I0840497

"When we first formed
People Incorporated,
we weren't sophisticated.
We had no experience.
But we knew one thing:

**If you keep
your eyes open,
doors open up."**

HARRY MAGHAKIAN
CO-FOUNDER
PEOPLE INCORPORATED

PEOPLE
INCORPORATED
MENTAL HEALTH SERVICES

THE FIRST 50

Opening Doors (Literally)

A pastor opens his church basement to a handful of veterans with mental and chemical health issues—and no place to go. We spend the next couple of decades swinging open doors on more than 20 programs helping people find their healthier, happier selves.

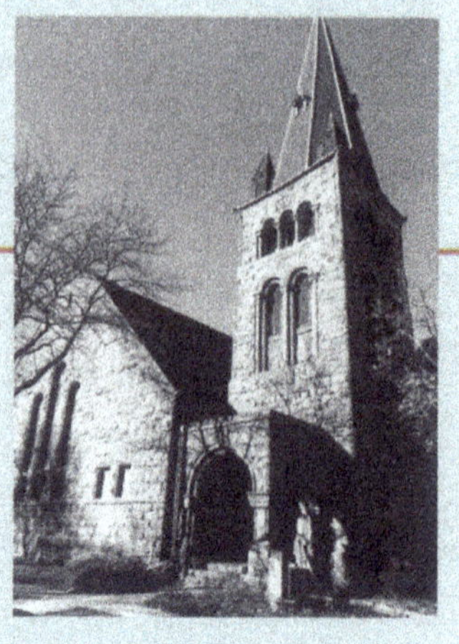

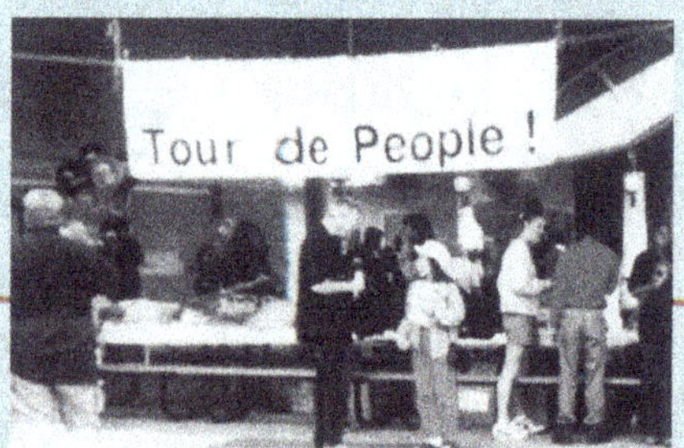

Open to Everything

It's the era of "Yes!" We're burgeoning with ideas on how to help build a mental health system where none existed before. Exploration, creation, innovation.

Open to a 360° View

Bring down the walls! We've spent 50 years inventing individual programs for specific needs of this vulnerable population. Now, we're shaping these programs into one full, open network of care—looking at every aspect of a person's life and helping where we can.

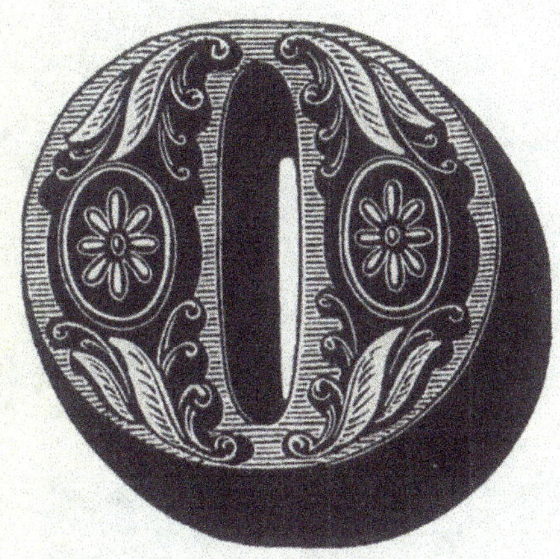

Once upon a time, back in the 1960s, state-run mental hospitals began shutting down.

The Theory: Patients would be less isolated and receive better treatment in community-based mental health services.

The Reality: There *weren't* many community-based mental health services!

So thousands of Minnesotans with mental illness were released to go—where exactly?

That's where our story begins.

The idea took root back in **1969**, in the Summit-University neighborhood of St. Paul, MN. **REV. HARRY MAGHAKIAN**, pastor at the Dayton Avenue Presbyterian Church, was troubled by the poverty and despair of his community. In particular, his big heart went out to the men living in the rooming house behind his church. Most of them had come out of the military suffering from **MENTAL ILLNESS.** To mask their symptoms, they were using **DRUGS AND ALCOHOL.**

Our Story

FROM THE GRASSROOTS UP

SYNOPSIS: They saw a need. Instead of stepping around it, they stepped in.

Harry invited them in off the streets to gather around the table in his **CHURCH BASEMENT.** Coffee, cookies, ashtrays, and a non-judgmental space kept the men coming back. Eventually, someone offered Harry a **GROUP HOME** as a gift, and the halfway house concept he'd been kicking around became real. **FOUR OTHER PASTORS** and their congregations joined Harry in his mission: **GEORGE KNIERIEMEN, JR.**, of North Como Presbyterian Church, **DON BUMP**, with the Merriam Lexington Presbyterian Church, **DAVID LING**, from the Presbyterian Church of the Way, and **HARRY SWEITZER**, of the Central Presbyterian Church.

This visionary team also included **PUBLIC SOCIAL WORKERS, JERROLD WINTERS** and **RONALD BOURDAGHS.**

THAT SAME YEAR, this group of concerned citizens officially became **PEOPLE, INCORPORATED.** (Yes! In the old days, the name included a comma!)

They opened **DAYTON HOUSE,** for 15 chemically dependent men. It was the very first of what would become a deep and diverse array of programs over the next half-century.

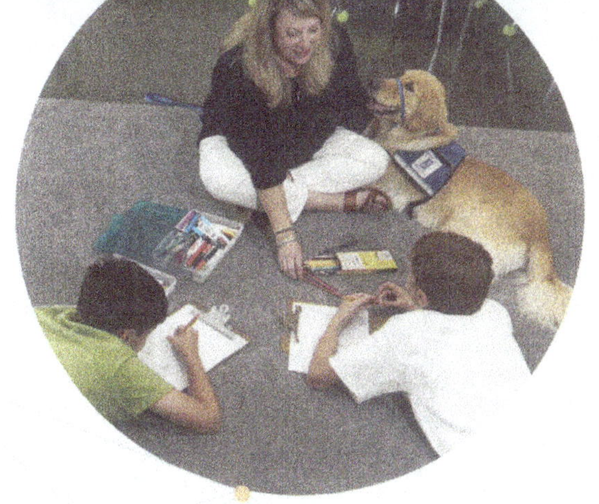

We have more than **700 STAFF**—and an infinite amount of passion—for helping people with mental illness find:

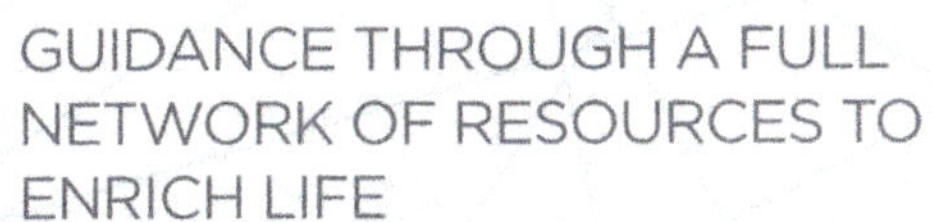

SAFE, SUPPORTIVE PLACES TO LIVE

GUIDANCE THROUGH A FULL NETWORK OF RESOURCES TO ENRICH LIFE

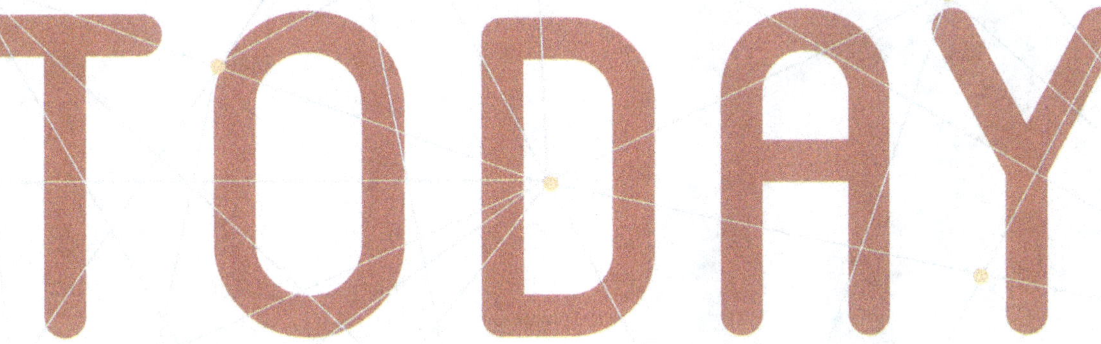

TODAY

We're the largest nonprofit community mental health provider in the Upper Midwest.

ASSISTANCE WHEN THEY HAVE NO HOME

THE CARE THEY NEED WHEN THEY'RE IN CRISIS

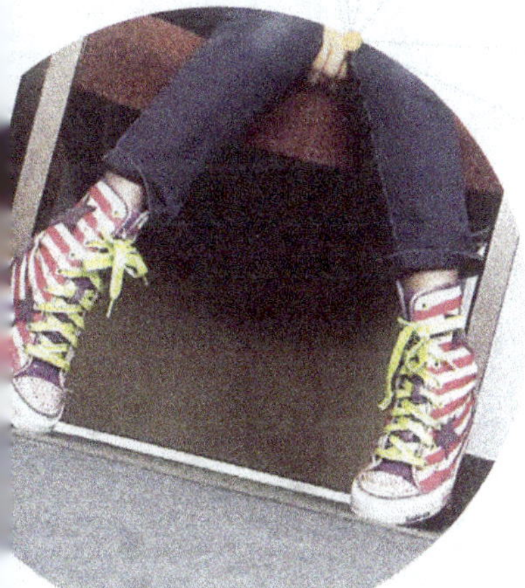

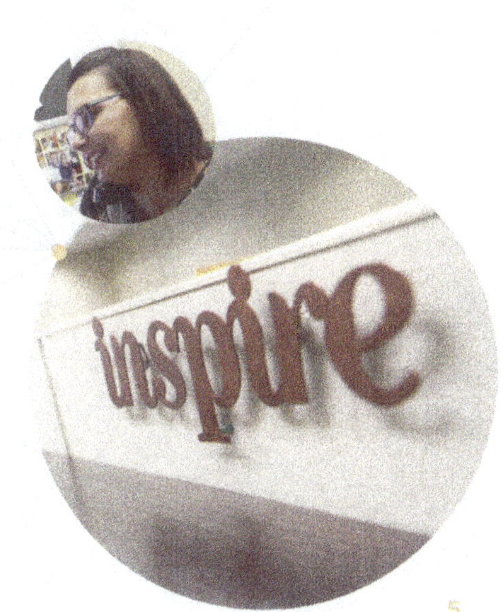

MENTAL AND PHYSICAL TREATMENT SERVICES

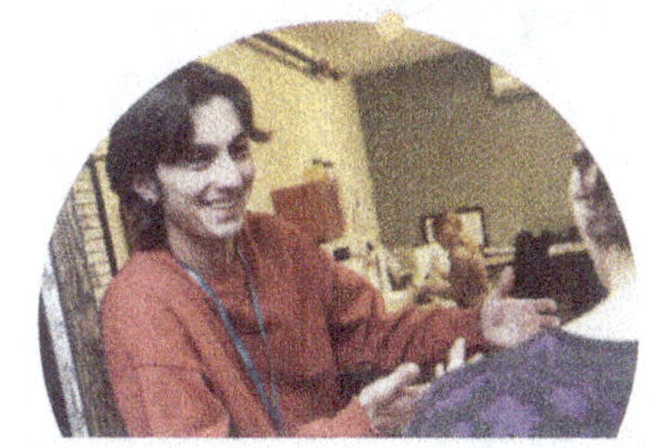

OPEN FOR REFUGE

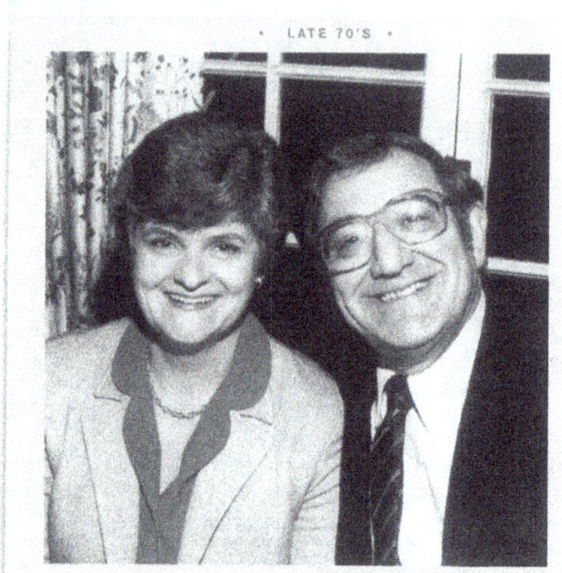

An excerpt from an interview with Harry and his wife, Judy

INTERVIEWER: *Why don't you start by talking about why you gravitated toward a life of service?*

JUDY: Part of Harry's sensitivity and awareness is that he's the child of immigrants. His parents came to this country and only spoke Armenian.

HARRY: I was born in this country, but my dad would say, "Բերանդ գոցէ, մեր խօսինք." In other words, "Don't forget. We are foreigners. Shut your mouth and be still."

JUDY: So being an immigrant, he understood what it meant to live on the margins. All of us, still today in the Armenian community, are called *odars*. An odar is an *outsider*. As an immigrant you're an outsider. And Harry tried to bring the outsiders in—into everything he did.

HARRY: And I think that's still very relevant. People Incorporated clients can feel like outsiders. They have lost their place.

Harry was a character preeminent. A well-intentioned guy, unrelenting, willing to tackle tough issues, not knowing where it was all going to go. But his DOOR WAS OPEN to everybody.

**PAUL VERRET
FINANCIAL SUPPORTER**

HARRY SAYS...

Barbara and Tim* would invite people to breakfast to educate them on People Incorporated. I would give the opening. I would put this on the center table, and I'd say, "What do you see?" When they took a good look at it, they'd discover it wasn't a left and a right hand. ***It was two right hands.***

It was two people together.

This statue is a reminder for us. That's the spirit of what's going on with People Incorporated.

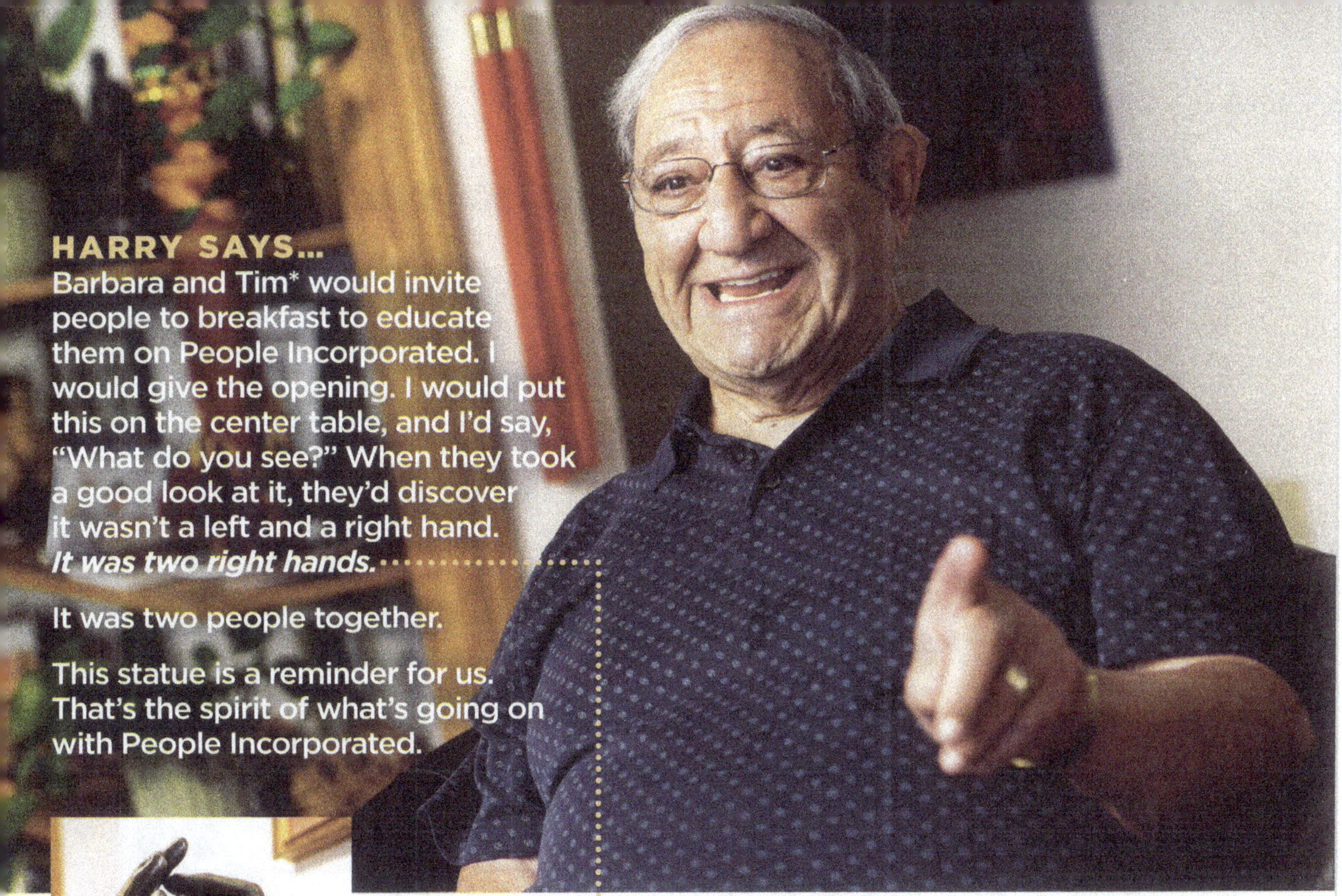

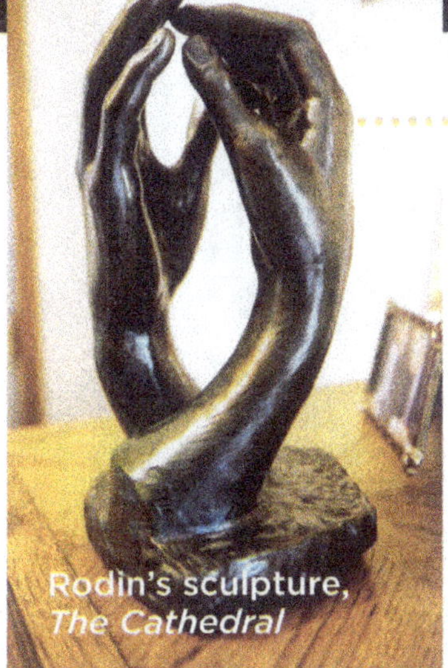

Rodin's sculpture, *The Cathedral*

What Harry did was really important. He took the first steps, and without a first step, you can't move forward.

JILL WIEDEMANN-WEST
CEO

INTERVIEWER: ***Is that how you came up with the name, People Incorporated—because you were incorporating people back into the community?***

HARRY: We were trying to give help and hope to those who had lost their connection. "Where is my home? Who can I lean on?"

So a few breakfasts after we got started, all of us were sitting around the table, and Harry Sweitzer** said, "People! We're talking about people!"

The name People Incorporated came up, and we said, "Hey, that fits!"

**VP of Community Relations, Barbara Nichols and Former CEO, Tim Burkett.*

***Harry Sweitzer was the pastor from Central Presbyterian, one of the five churches that founded People Incorporated.*

" HARRY MAGHAKIAN WAS CONSIDERED THE MONEY GUY. THAT'S WHAT DAD SAID—HE COULD JUST REACH INTO A DRAWER AND FIND MONEY!

SUE LITECKY, DAUGHTER OF ORIGINAL BOARD MEMBER, FRANK STAFFENSON

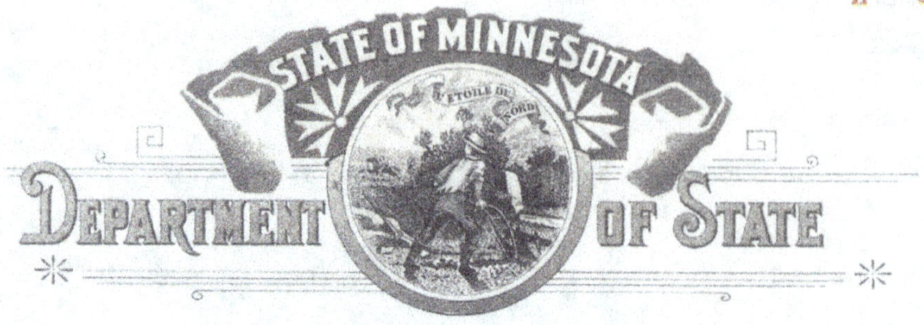

To All To Whom These Presents Shall Come, Greeting:

Whereas, Articles of Incorporation, duly signed and acknowledged under oath, have been recorded in the office of the Secretary of State, on the __--1st--__ day of __July__, A. D. 19_69_ for the incorporation of

__People, Incorporated__

under and in accordance with the provisions of the Minnesota Nonprofit Corporation Act, Minnesota Statutes, Chapter 317;

Now, Therefore, I, Joseph L. Donovan, Secretary of State of the State of Minnesota, by virtue of the powers and duties vested in me by law, do hereby certify that the said

__People, Incorporated__

is a legally organized Corporation under the laws of this State.

Witness my official signature hereunto subscribed and the Great Seal of the State of Minnesota hereunto affixed this __--first--__ day of __July__ in the year of our Lord one thousand nine hundred and __sixty-nine__

Joseph L. Donovan
Secretary of State.

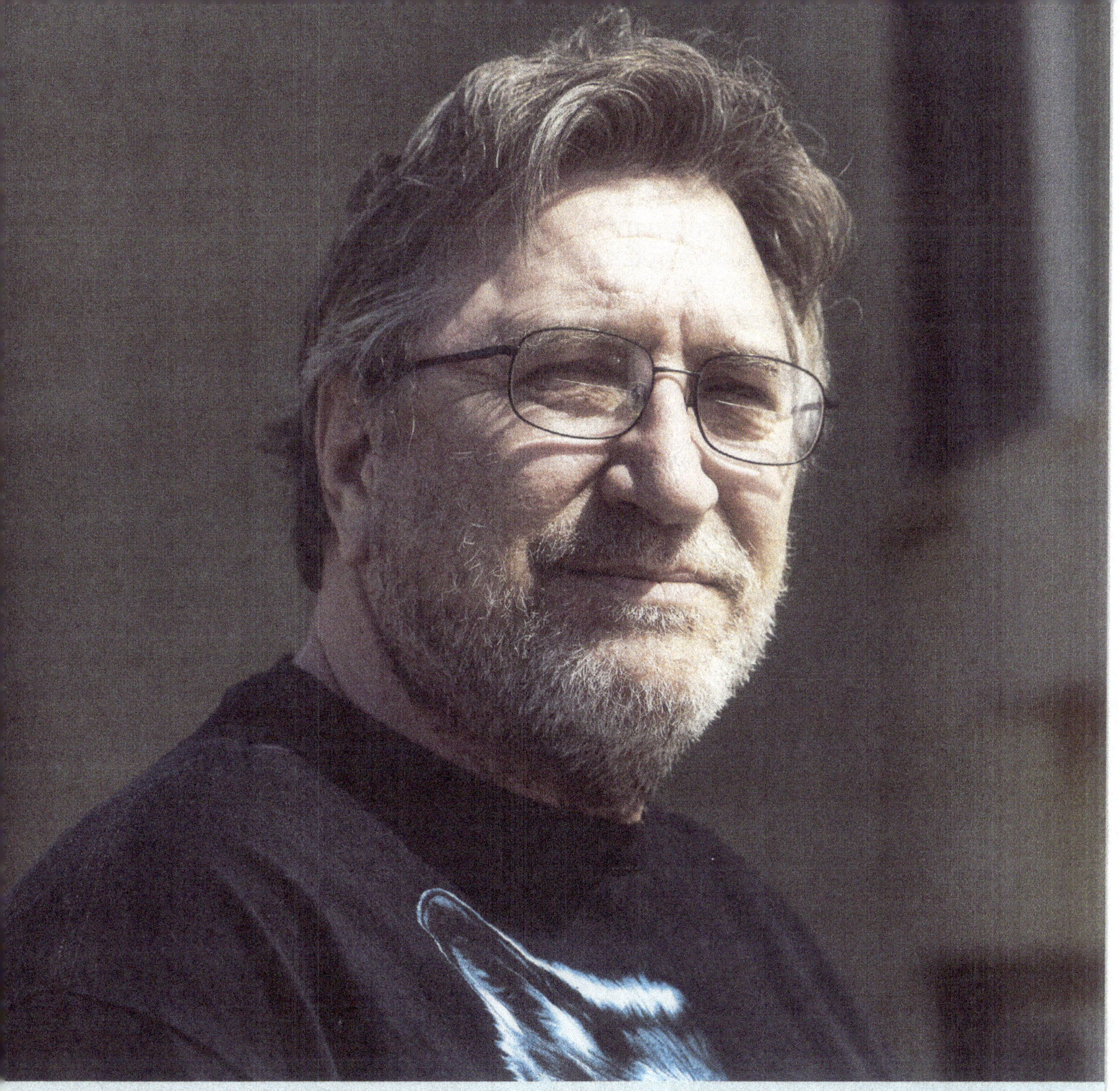

MEET RANDY.

He woke up one day in a ditch by the
freeway. He'd been waving his handmade
sign at drivers coming off the exit ramp.

Today, he's an author.

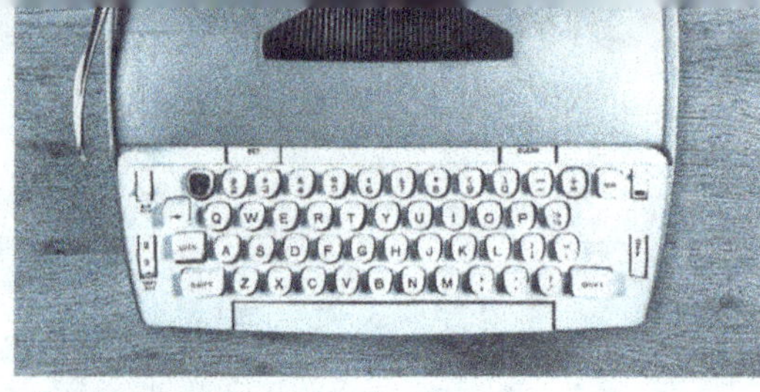

In the very beginning, maybe up until '77 or '78, we couldn't afford anything. We had to bring in our own typewriters, adding machines, pens, and pencils to work. Some of the people who worked for 3M would make a copy machine available to us so we could make copies.

DON BUMP, FORMER EXECUTIVE DIRECTOR

One of the things that we needed was a bus. Do you know how we got it? The women at the Presbyterian Church of the Twin Cities quickly collected enough Green Stamps to get us a bus. It was people involved with people.

**JUDY MAGHAKIAN,
WIFE OF CO-FOUNDER,
HARRY MAGHAKIAN**

The Hard

We were having a hard time making payroll. I called up the county, and I said, "Listen. People Incorporated is about to go down for the third time." They called me in. And when I came down to the meeting—and it chokes me up even today—every department head in the county was there. It was like—holy crap! We got support from them, from day one.

**GLENN ANDERSON
FORMER EXECUTIVE DIRECTOR**

(AUTHOR'S NOTE: Yup. Glenn was choking up when he told us this story.).....

WE HAD ONE FINANCE PERSON WHO WANTED US TO KEEP COUNT OF THE ROLLS OF TOILET PAPER.

**MARY KAY MCJILTON
VICE PRESIDENT**

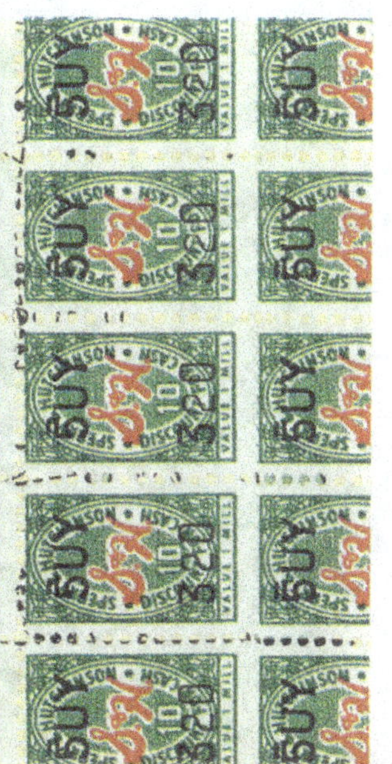

We were slapping it together. We didn't have the money in the bank. We didn't have power and so on. So consequently, you did what you had to do today for tomorrow. We didn't look down the road any further than that. And now when People Incorporated boastfully says they serve 10,000 people, they're doing it responsibly, and we can applaud.

Old Days

The financial basis was very, very shaky. People Incorporated was a real boost for my faith, because we did some things on faith alone!!

**DIANE E. FOLLMER
BOARD MEMBER, 1970**

Back in the old days—maybe in the 80s?—my boss and I would work all day, and then in the evenings we'd sell pull tabs at a bar! We didn't make squat, but we were trying to raise funds. We used to hold plant sales, too.

PAM, BILLING SPECIALIST

People Incorporated never told me during my job interviews that the agency was actually bankrupt. Insolvent, anyway. I walked in the door on my first day of work, and that's when I found out.

**GLENN ANDERSON
FORMER EXECUTIVE DIRECTOR**

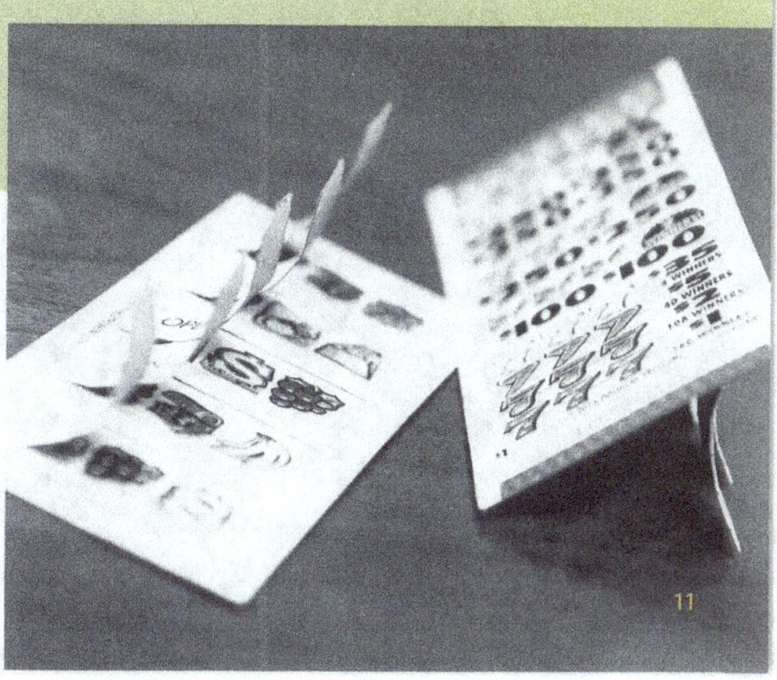

Supporting mental health AND WELLNESS in our community *through collaboration* AND INTEGRATION OF CARE

THOSE WERE PROBABLY THE WORST DAYS OF MY LIFE.

"When taking another breath seemed impossible because the darkness was just so overwhelming. But no matter how deep down I got, they were always kind. **I THINK WITHOUT THE STAFF AT PEOPLE INCORPORATED I WOULD NOT BE HERE. I WOULD HAVE DIED.**"

MELANIE, CLIENT

Employees can donate money to a fund for client needs.

"Once I remember buying a suit and a bus ticket for a client so he could go to his father's funeral in Chicago. Another time we sent a Native American woman to a Pow Wow. It shows how much the staff really believes in the mission."

JOAN, PROGRAM DIRECTOR

Last year staff contributed
$18,212
to the Client Needs Fund.

"To be able to go to the **APOLLO DROP-IN CENTER*** — that place was just magical. When you have mental illness, it's hard to find somewhere you feel like you belong. **HAVING A PLACE WHERE THEY LET YOU STAY ISN'T THE SAME AS HAVING A PLACE WHERE YOU BELONG.**"

PETE, CLIENT

We've embedded a clinical social worker in the St. Paul Police Department.

"I'm extremely grateful to People Incorporated. After we de-escalate a mental health situation, we now have someone with us to offer a long-term solution for the person in crisis. Lives are being changed."

**SERGEANT JAMIE SIPES
ST. PAUL POLICE DEPT.**

Jan's daughter had mental illness. Before finding People Incorporated, the family struggled with their treatment experience.

"We were so blown away by how disjointed the service provision was for our daughter. She'd have a counselor, and then she'd have a psychiatrist. And then she'd be hospitalized. She'd be released, and there'd be no communication with the person who was going to see her next. We just struggled to know how to help her through that maze."

**JAN ANDERSON
FORMER BOARD CHAIR**

**Our Apollo Resource Center was a place where people with mental illness came to hang out, support one another, and access other resources on a drop-in basis.*

13

What do we have?
STIGMA

It makes people with mental
illness feel lonely and isolated.

WE'RE NOT WHERE WE NEED TO BE YET.
It takes time for a human rights movement to take hold.

SUE ABDERHOLDEN, NATIONAL ALLIANCE ON MENTAL ILLNESS (NAMI)

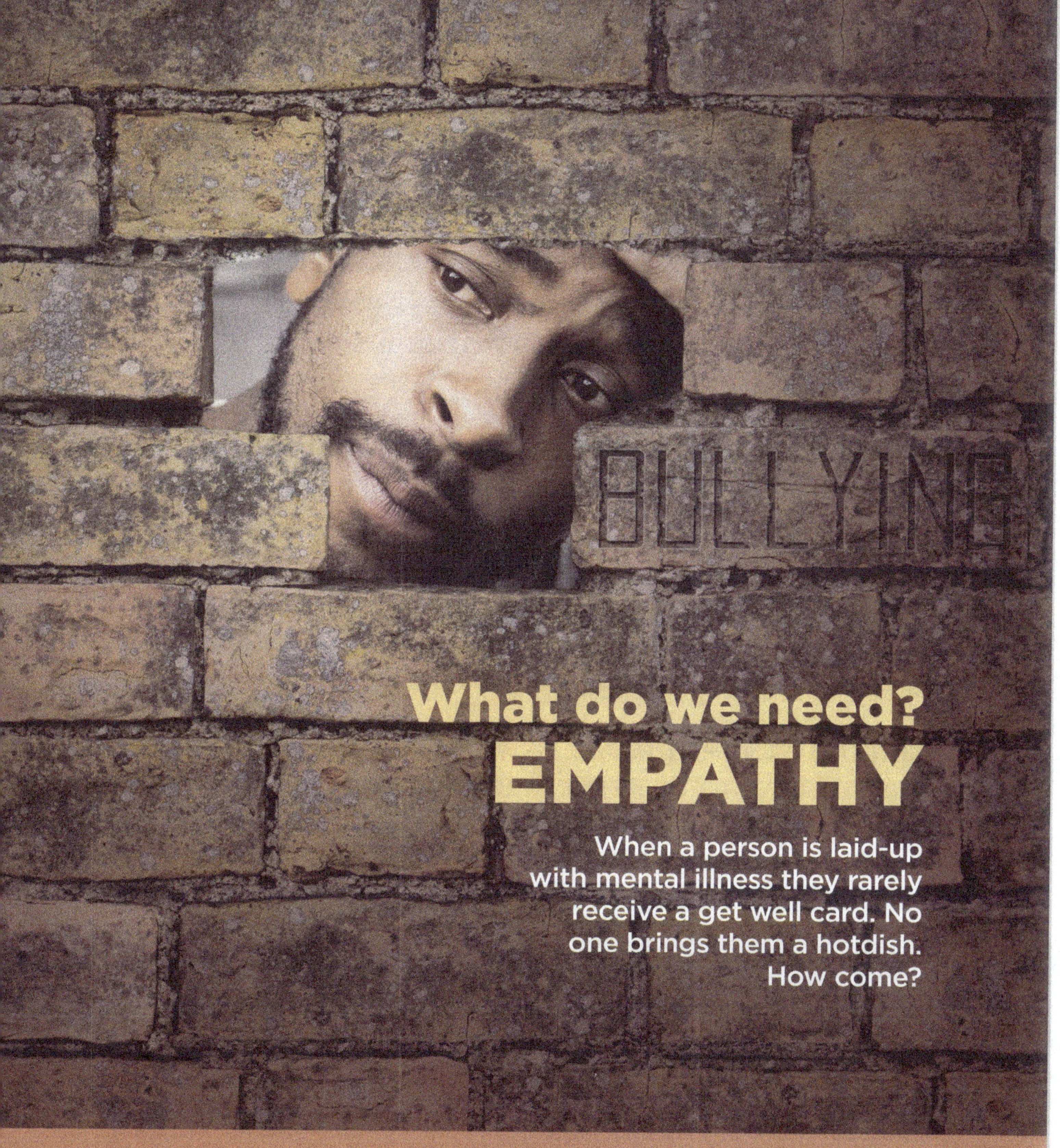
BULLYING

What do we need?
EMPATHY

When a person is laid-up
with mental illness they rarely
receive a get well card. No
one brings them a hotdish.
How come?

We should be ashamed as a nation that
OVER 100 PEOPLE TAKE THEIR OWN LIVES EVERY DAY.
JILL WIEDEMANN-WEST, CEO

We try to stay

PERSON-CENTERED

in every conversation with our clients.

We find out what they want from life
and shine a light in that direction.

Let's say a client really wants a job in the community. Our role would be to help her break that down into attainable, realistic goals: Maybe she'd want to focus on taking her medications on schedule. That could help her get out of bed on time—which a job would require.

MELISSA, SENIOR PROGRAM MANAGER

It's about the individual themselves. It's like, we know I cannot fix or carry you, but you can fix and carry yourself. So how can I walk with you down that path?

ALBERT, PEER SUPPORT SPECIALIST

Being person-centered means balancing what's important *to* somebody with what's important *for* them.

Is the idea of person-centered care new to People Incorporated?

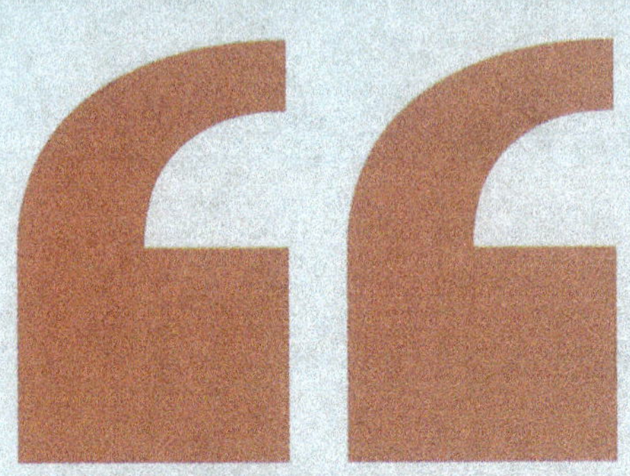

A church will tell someone what they need. Baloney! **YOU DON'T TELL THEM WHAT THEY NEED. YOU LISTEN.** And then you create programs around that. There's a world of difference in that approach. And we used that approach in everything we did.

JUDY MAGHAKIAN, HARRY'S WIFE

A day-treatment client at Children's Services wrote to staff member, Pam.

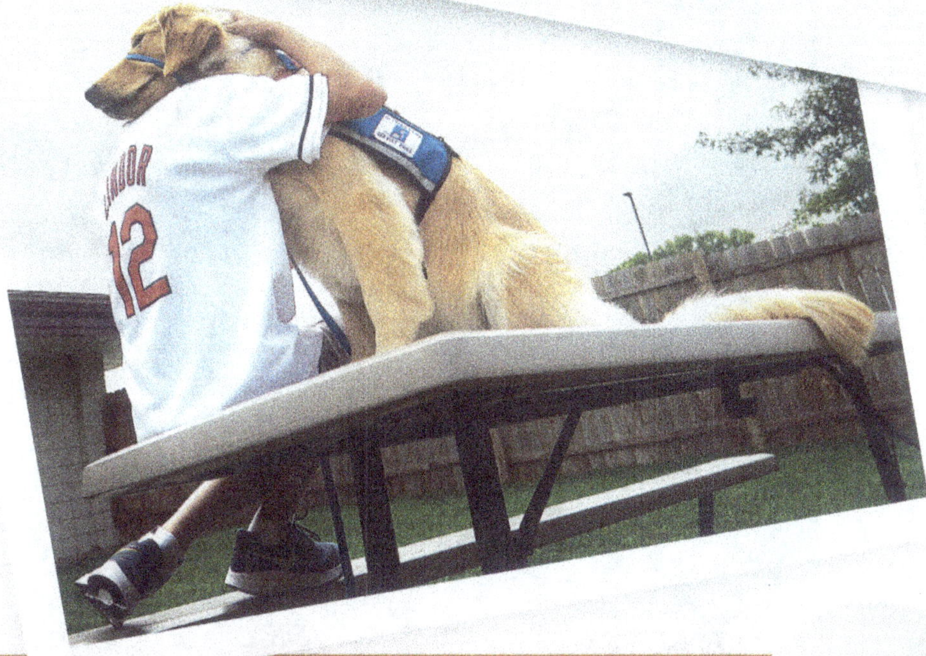

Canine staff member, AJ, is specially trained to help kids feel calm and relaxed.

I used to work in the schools, and kids were given up on pretty quickly if they had behavior outbursts. But here we create a sense of hope in the kids. They can mess up, but we're still going to care about them.

It's part of the PERSON-CENTERED APPROACH. Being friendly, being nurturing. Helping them make a change.

PAM, SENIOR PROGRAM MANAGER

JUST THINK

HALF OF ALL CHRONIC MENTAL ILLNESS BEGINS BY AGE 14

Intervening with kids right away can change their patterns, help them think differently, and lower the negative impact on their lives.

QUESTION:
What causes mental illness?

ANSWER:
That depends. What year is it?

4000 YEARS AGO

CAUSE:
A woman's uterus wanders to another part of her body

CURE:
Strong-smelling substances lure it back into place

1500 YEARS AGO

CAUSE:
Demonic possession

CURE:
A hole drilled into the skull lets evil spirits out

500 YEARS AGO

CAUSE:
Mental illness is a choice

CURE:
Threats, electric shock, induced-vomiting, ice-water baths, bloodletting

250 YEARS AGO

CAUSE:
Poor distribution of magnetic fluid in the body

CURE:
Iron rods attached to the body redistribute the fluid

80 YEARS AGO

CAUSE:
Repressed memories

CURE:
Getting patient to recall memories

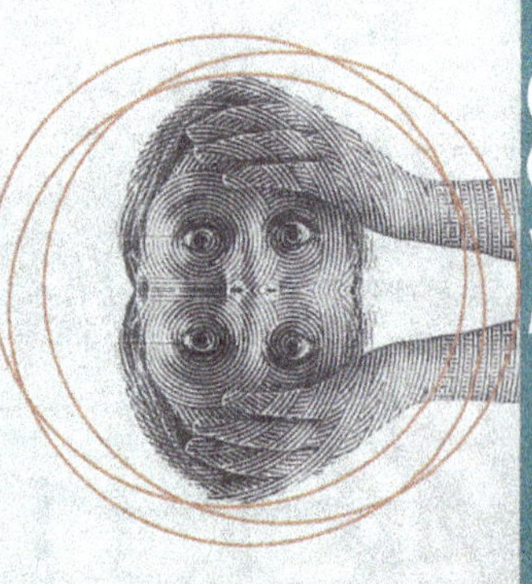

HERE'S THE TRUTH:
We still don't know the truth.
A mental health condition is probably the result of multiple, linking causes including factors like genetics, lifestyle, biochemistry, environment, and brain structure.

Leaps and Bounds

Effective **ANTIPSYCHOTIC MEDS** introduced

The American Medical Association defines addiction to **ALCOHOL AND DRUGS AS A DISEASE**

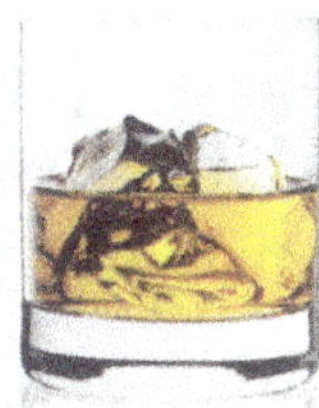

BEHAVIOR THERAPY becomes widespread

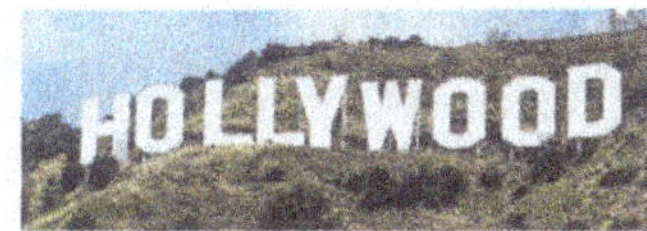

The film release of ***ONE FLEW OVER THE CUCKOO'S NEST*** causes mistrust of—and improvements to—mental health treatment

More effective antipsychotic meds with **FEWER SIDE EFFECTS** become available

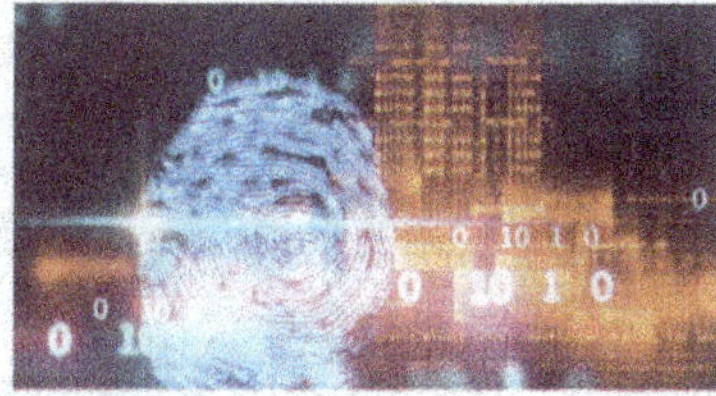

Care options are driven by **HIGHER-QUALITY DATA**

1950s

1960s

1970s

1980s

1990s

2006

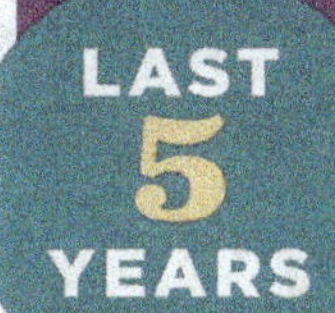

ASYLUMS ARE SHUTTING DOWN at an alarming rate, forcing patients out— and often into homelessness

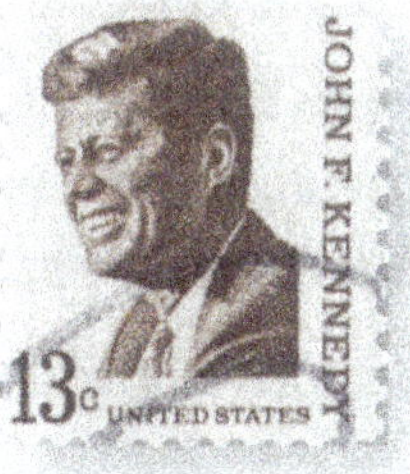

President Kennedy signs an act to fund construction of more **COMMUNITY-BASED TREATMENT FACILITIES**

New and **BETTER ANTIDEPRESSANTS** are introduced

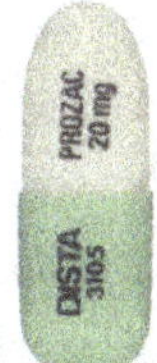

There's a push to build a **COMMUNITY NETWORK OF CARE**

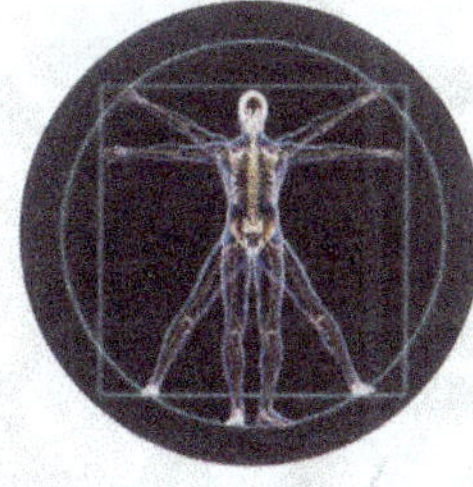

THE WHOLE-PERSON APPROACH to care emerges (addressing mental, physical, and social aspects)

Efforts to **FILL GAPS** in the mental health care system continue

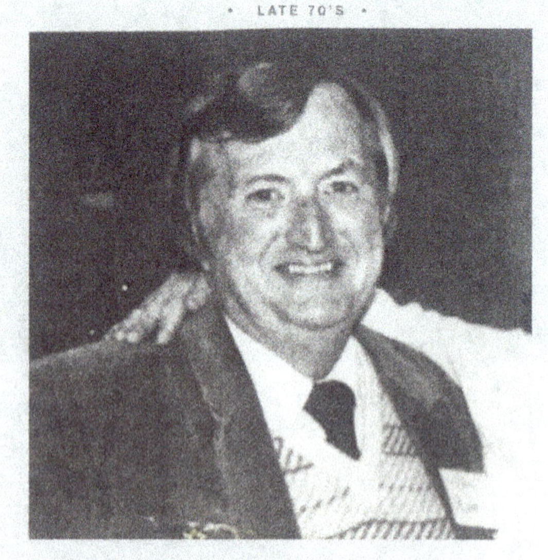

OPEN TO

An excerpt from an interview with Don

INTERVIEWER: *You were the first Executive Director at People Incorporated, right?*

DON: Well, they hired a man (named Larry Granger) in 1972, but he resigned after a year. So I took the job in 1974 and stayed for 12 years.

INTERVIEWER: *You must have liked the work.*

DON: I fell in love with the corporation. The church was not sitting in judgment, saying, "Oh, you're going to Hell if you don't straighten out." They were saying, "It's not about where you'll go if you don't get treatment—it's where you'll go if you do. The sky's the limit, and we'll help you get there."

INTERVIEWER: *Back in those early days, People Incorporated had all kinds of programs—not just those for mental illness. Do any stand out for you?*

One day we got a call from a group that had a program for physically and developmentally disabled children. The state was threatening to close it, so they asked us to take it over.

That one really gripped my heart. Our staff was just so darn good. I mean, they were able to cry with the kids, and laugh with the kids, and challenge the kids.

Don Bump really carried the ball as the first Executive Director. During his tenure, there were a whole bunch of programs he created that already existed when I showed up.

GLENN ANDERSON,
FORMER EXECUTIVE DIRECTOR

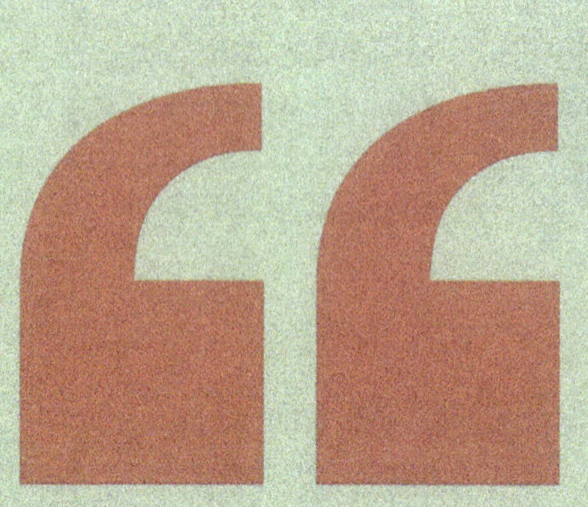

THERE WERE JUST SO MANY SITUATIONS WHERE WE NEEDED HELP FROM KEY PEOPLE IN THE COMMUNITY. They gave us their time, their energy, and their love. And when they needed help, we'd open doors for them as well.

—DON BUMP, EXECUTIVE DIRECTOR, 1974–1986

COLLABORATION

 What else makes you feel emotional when you think back on those days?

That's easy. **THE BOARD OF DIRECTORS.** ....
They were willing to take chances. They were willing to stick their necks out. I could go to them with anything. Anything! They were always open.

" DON HAD THE HEART. AND A LOT OF KNOWLEDGE.

HARRY MAGHAKIAN, CO-FOUNDER

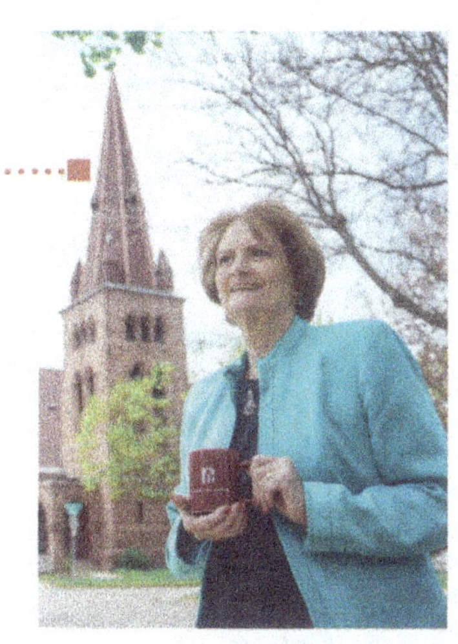

HISTORY BIT

Diane E. Follmer is one of the early board members Don is talking about. In fact, she holds the record for longest-serving board member, with a whopping 26 years!

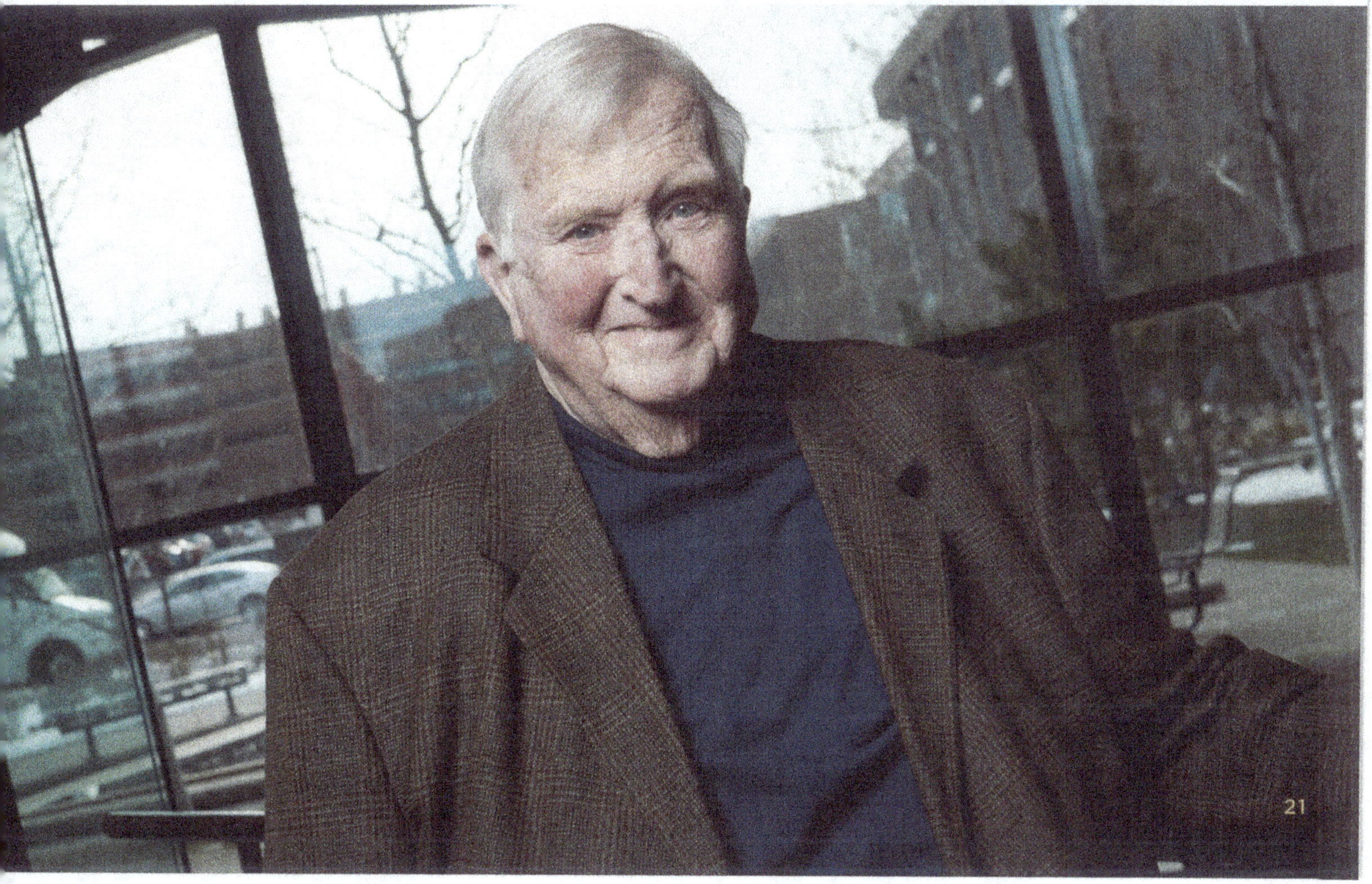

THE FIRST RESIDENTIAL PROGRAM IN THE U.S. FOR PEOPLE WHO ARE DEAF OR HARD OF HEARING AND HAVE MENTAL ILLNESS

Great American Cowboys

Fighting for the Deaf and Hard of Hearing

People with severe or total hearing loss had no residential mental health resource.

Until the People Incorporated Cowboys rode into town.

From MARY KAY MCJILTON VICE PRESIDENT:

We opened a program for the deaf—in this elegant, modern house, with neighbors who weren't thrilled about us being there. A woman from Hennepin County came out, and she said, "My god, all this glass. We've heard about these volatile deaf people. They're going to break every window."

They never broke a thing, of course.

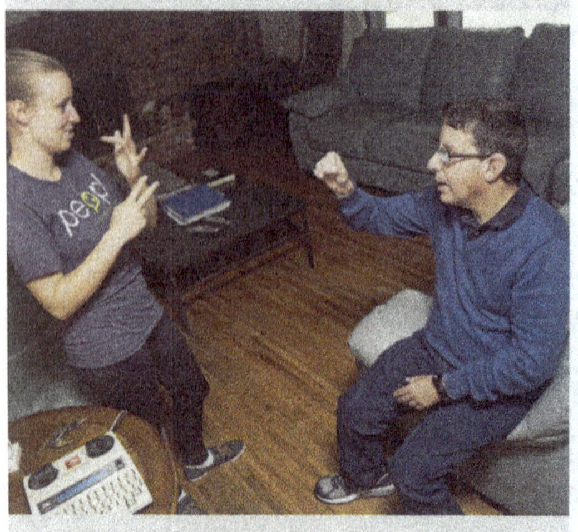

So there were some hitches in the git-along at first. But a cowboy climbs into the saddle ready to ride.

From GLENN ANDERSON, FORMER EXECUTIVE DIRECTOR:

It was very unique because all the staff were deaf. The very idea of providing mental health services to deaf people was an interesting adventure and culture clash.

One day we had a psycho-pharmacology training session. Two sign language interpreters were explaining all the psychotropic medications for different diagnoses. There was no ASL sign for phenothiazine, right? So they were finger spelling to the point where they came up to me after the meeting and said, "Don't ever ask us to do that again."

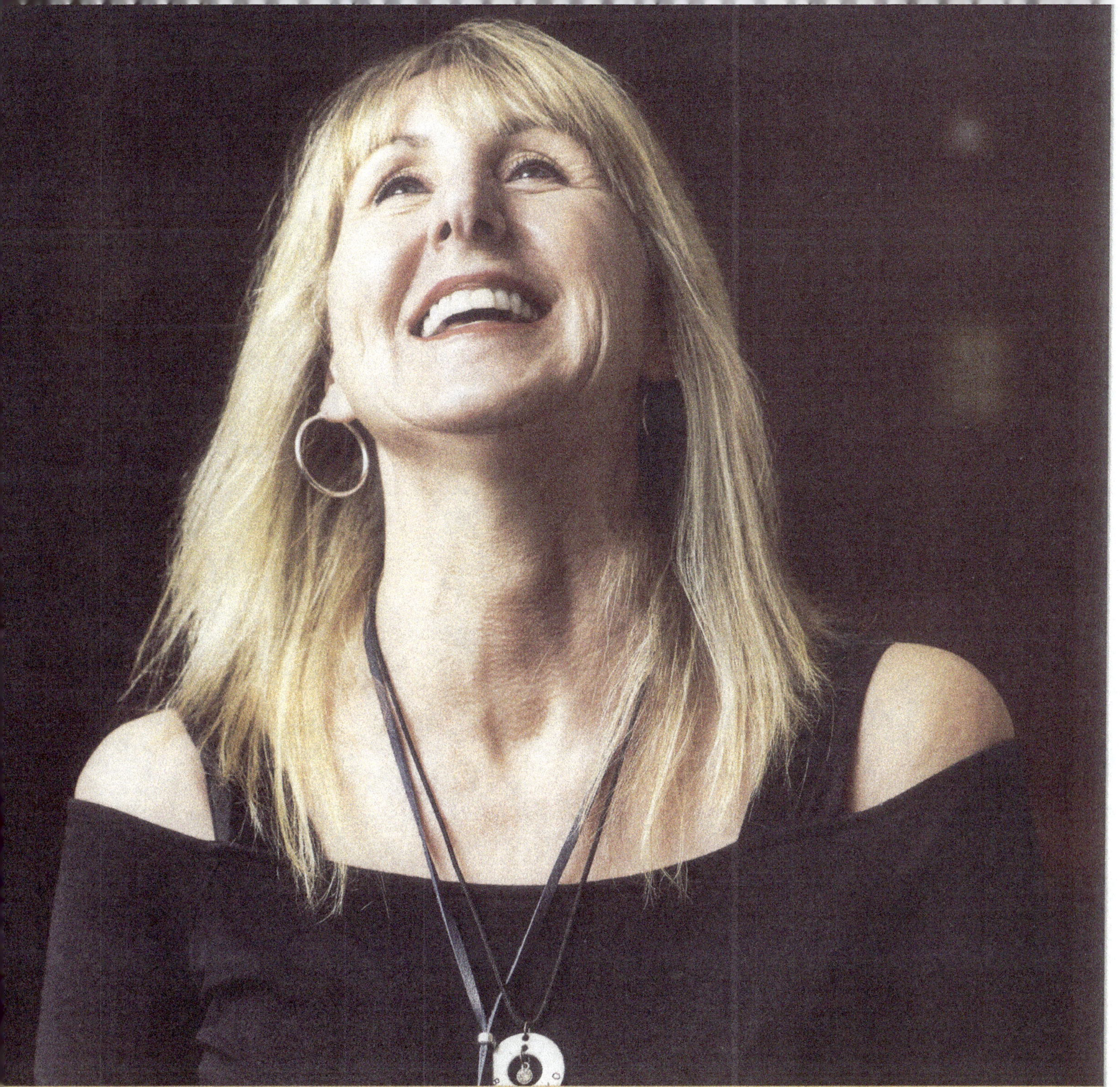

MEET KATHLEEN.

She woke up crying—or screaming—
every morning for weeks.

*Today she has an infectious laugh
and a plan to raise chickens.*

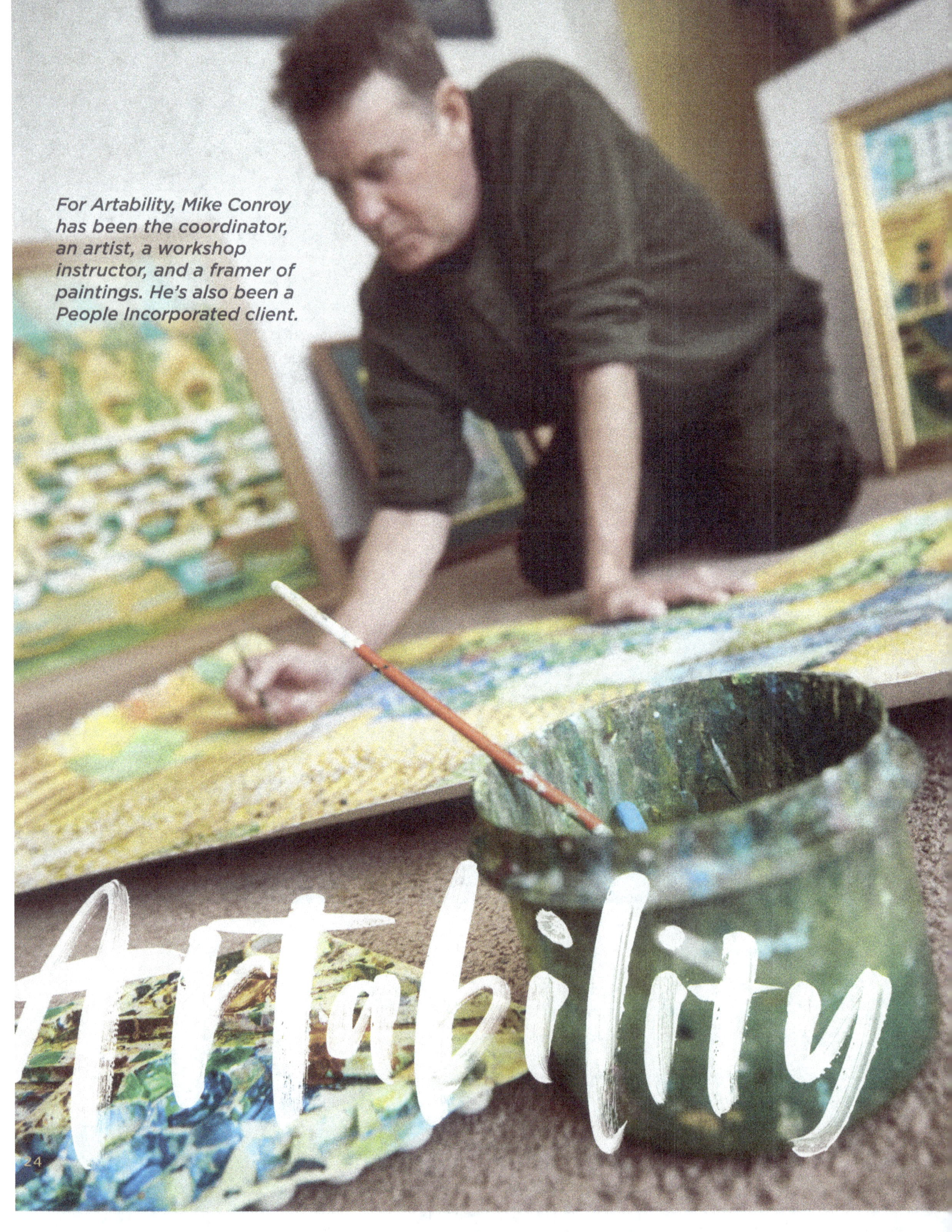
For Artability, Mike Conroy
has been the coordinator,
an artist, a workshop
instructor, and a framer of
paintings. He's also been a
People Incorporated client.
Artability

ART meets **party** meets **"LOOK AT THAT!"** meets **self-expression** meets **life experience. That's Artability.**

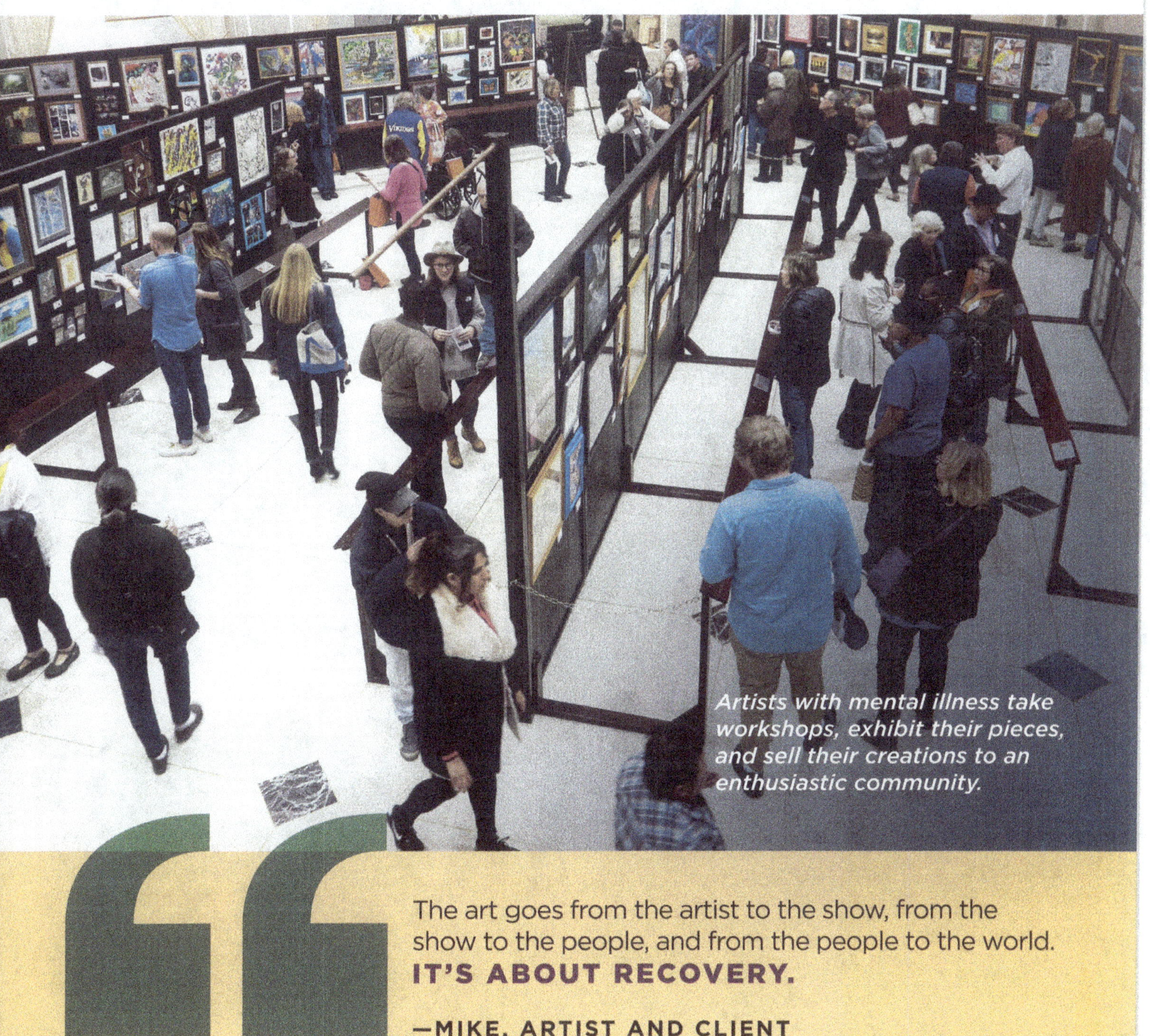

> The art goes from the artist to the show, from the show to the people, and from the people to the world. **IT'S ABOUT RECOVERY.**
>
> **—MIKE, ARTIST AND CLIENT**

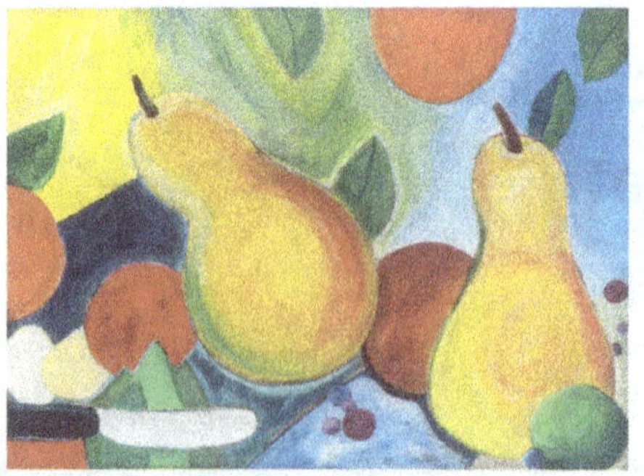

Gail Harbeck, *Pears*

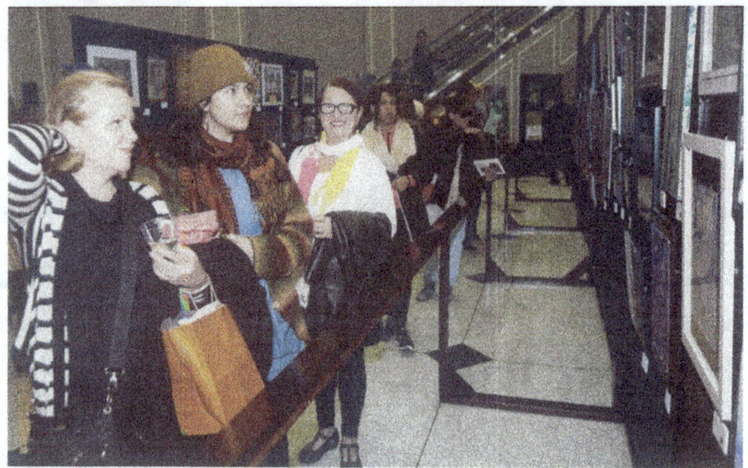

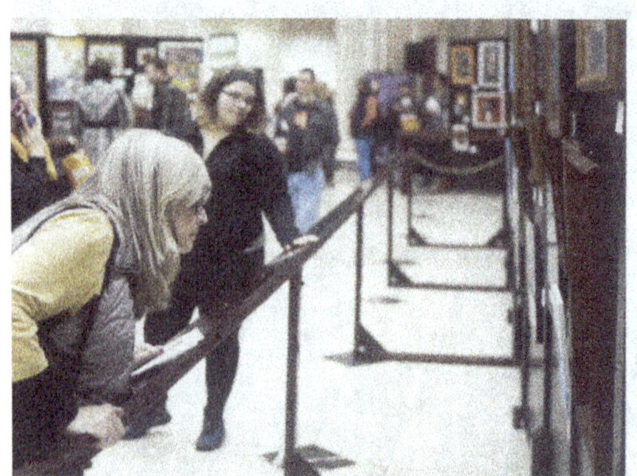

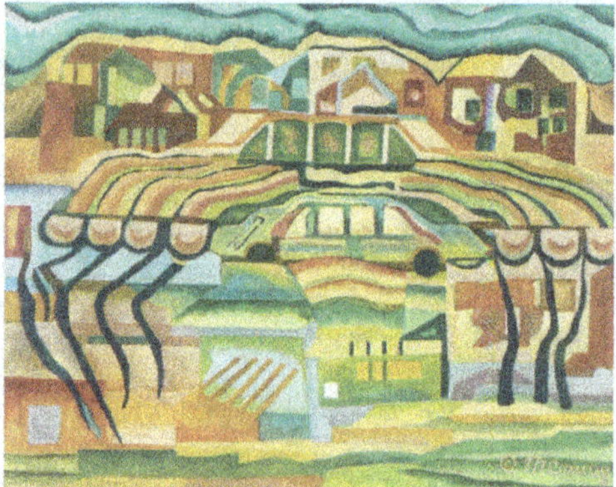

Michael Conroy, *Superior Handling*

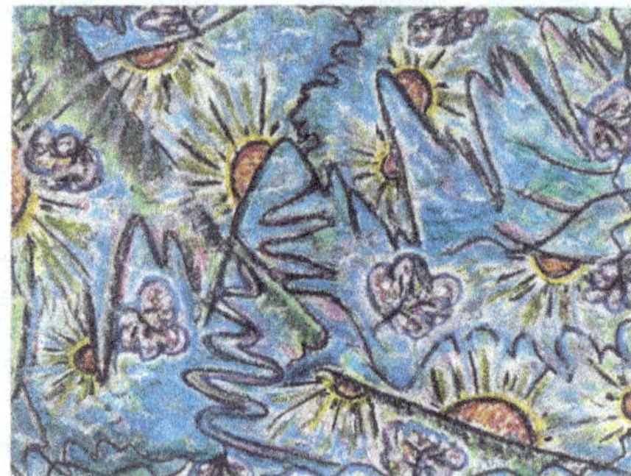

Laurie Nelson, *Sunrises*

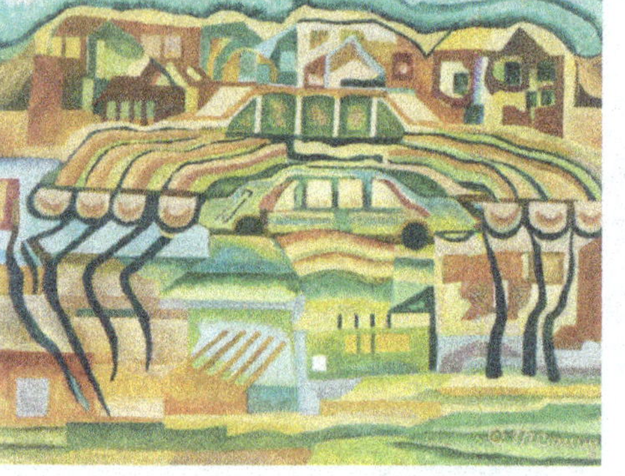

Shining Starr, *Starr's Fantasia*

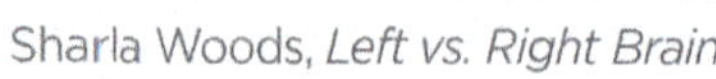

Sharla Woods, *Left vs. Right Brain*

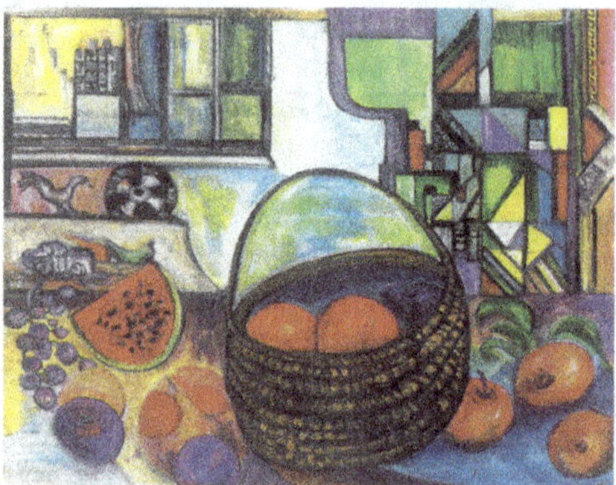

Faye Buffington-Howell,
A Basket of Opportunities

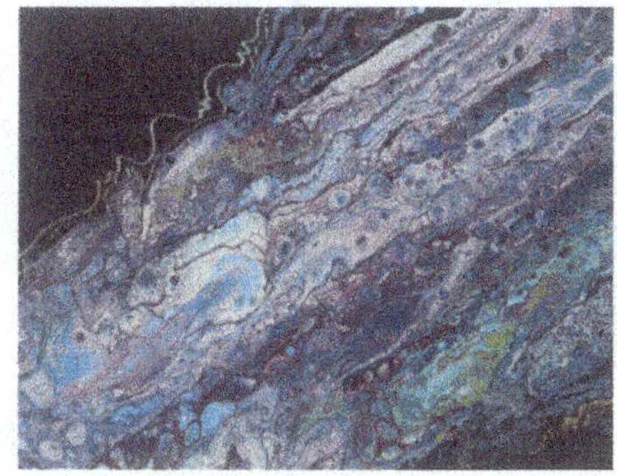

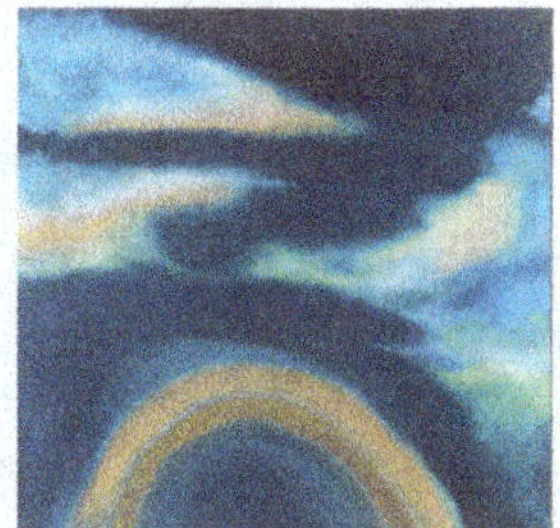

Karen Wood, *Strömma*

Marcia Berge, *Dusk*

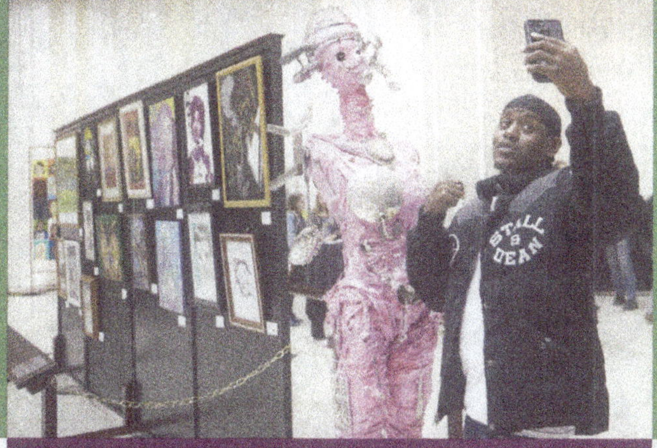

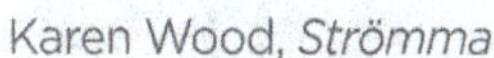

It began in the late 1990s, at our APOLLO Resource Center. A few clients had displayed their paintings in the form of an art show for family and friends.

THEN THIS PERSON CAME ALONG.

Barbara Nichols saw the potential to turn this intimate activity into a life-altering event.

Expanding Artability was just one of the ways Barbara helped People Incorporated win hearts in the community. The year before she came on staff, the organization had brought in only $4400 from donors. Over the next 16 years, Barbara would help raise, in total, more than 23 million dollars from donors, corporations, and foundations.

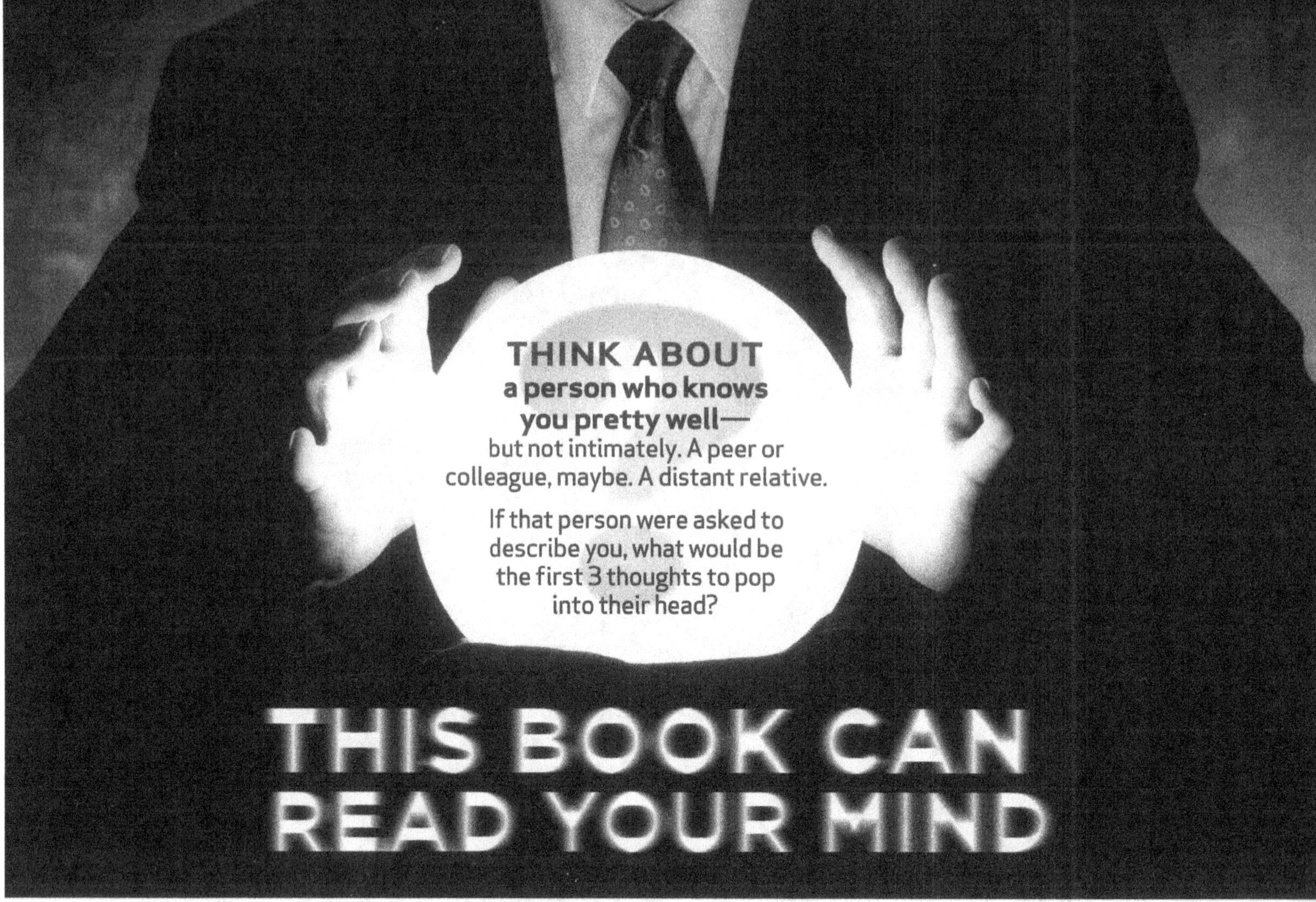

THE CRYSTAL BALL SAYS...

MAGGIE IS A BRILLIANT PIANIST WITH PURPLE EYES WHO RIDES A VINTAGE MOTORCYCLE. BUT EVERYONE AT WORK SEES HER AS THE LADY WHO COULDN'T GET OUT OF BED FOR A MONTH.

IF you don't have a misunderstood disability (*like mental illness*), you responded with one or more of these:

- A physical aspect (*e.g. red hair, Japanese*)
- A role you fill (*e.g. neighbor, computer geek*)
- A personality trait (*e.g. funny, brainiac*)
- A unique behavior (*e.g. reads in the park, walks fast*)

BUT IF you do have a misunderstood disability (*like mental illness*), it was on the list.

HOW DID THE CRYSTAL BALL KNOW? The idea of mental illness can make people uncomfortable, so it's a trait that stands out. It often leads to a person getting defined by their illness.

Freud talks about a healthy individual as someone who can LOVE and WORK.

I would add to that a person who can PLAY.

LOVE is how you feel connected.

WORK is where you feel meaningful.

PLAY makes life feel like it's worth living.

—*Tim McGuire*
Director of
Quality Assurance

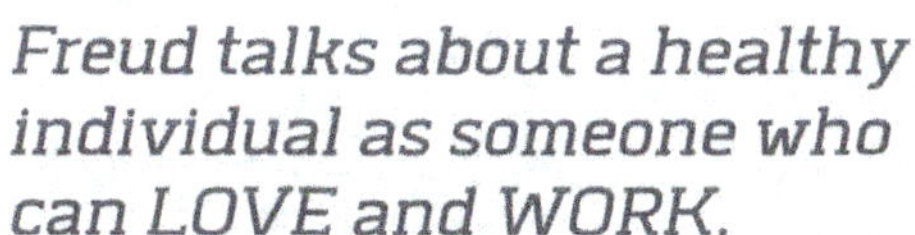

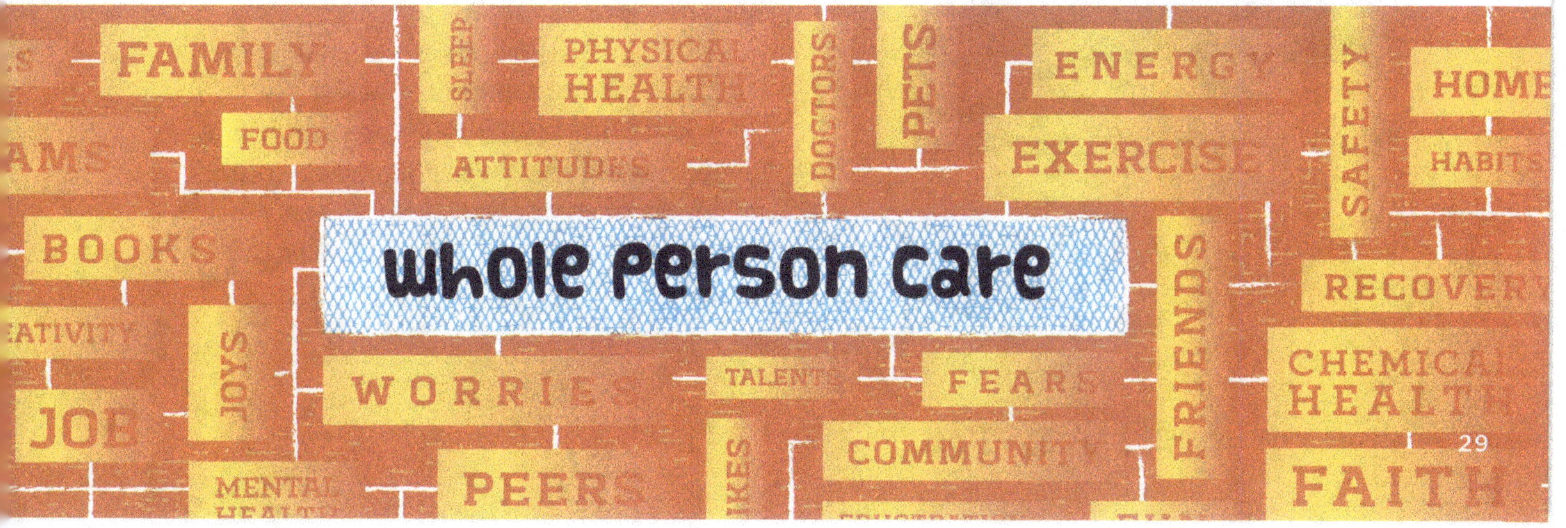

An excerpt from an interview with Glenn

INTERVIEWER: *Looking back, what type of leader were you?*

GLENN: What came to my mind just now was a spark plug. I was the one who wanted to do all the stuff that I had to talk everybody else into.

People would worry. "What if it doesn't work?"

And I'd say, "Then we'll try something else."

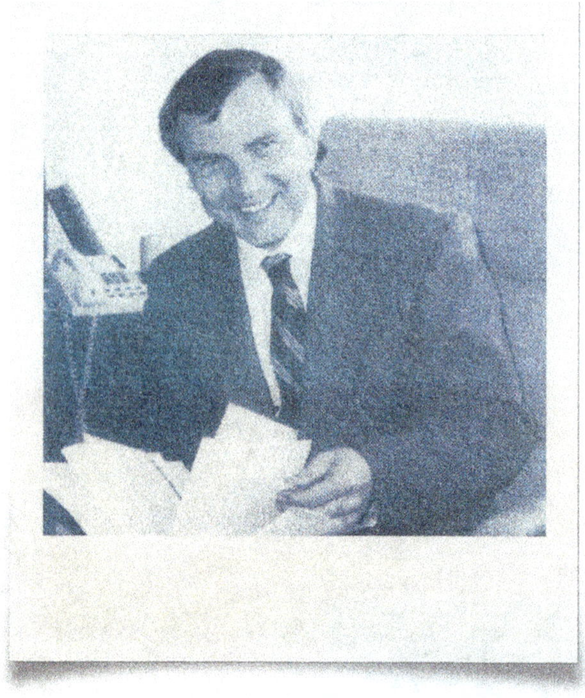

INTERVIEWER: *Try something like starting a community support and housing program for people with epilepsy?*

GLENN: Right. We were asked, so we did it. I'm sort of like a guy with his hair on fire. Completely reckless. My theory was—and is—never pass up an opportunity.

INTERVIEWER: *But epilepsy? It isn't a mental illness.*

GLENN: No, but People Incorporated wasn't that picky back in those days. Originally, mental illness wasn't even on the list.

OPEN TO

INTERVIEWER: *It sounds like this was a pretty thrilling time in your life.*

GLENN: It was a righteous adventure. I mean, the question was always, "Okay, what kind of service model would meet this particular need? Let's take out a blank sheet of paper and write down what it should look like, and let's do that."

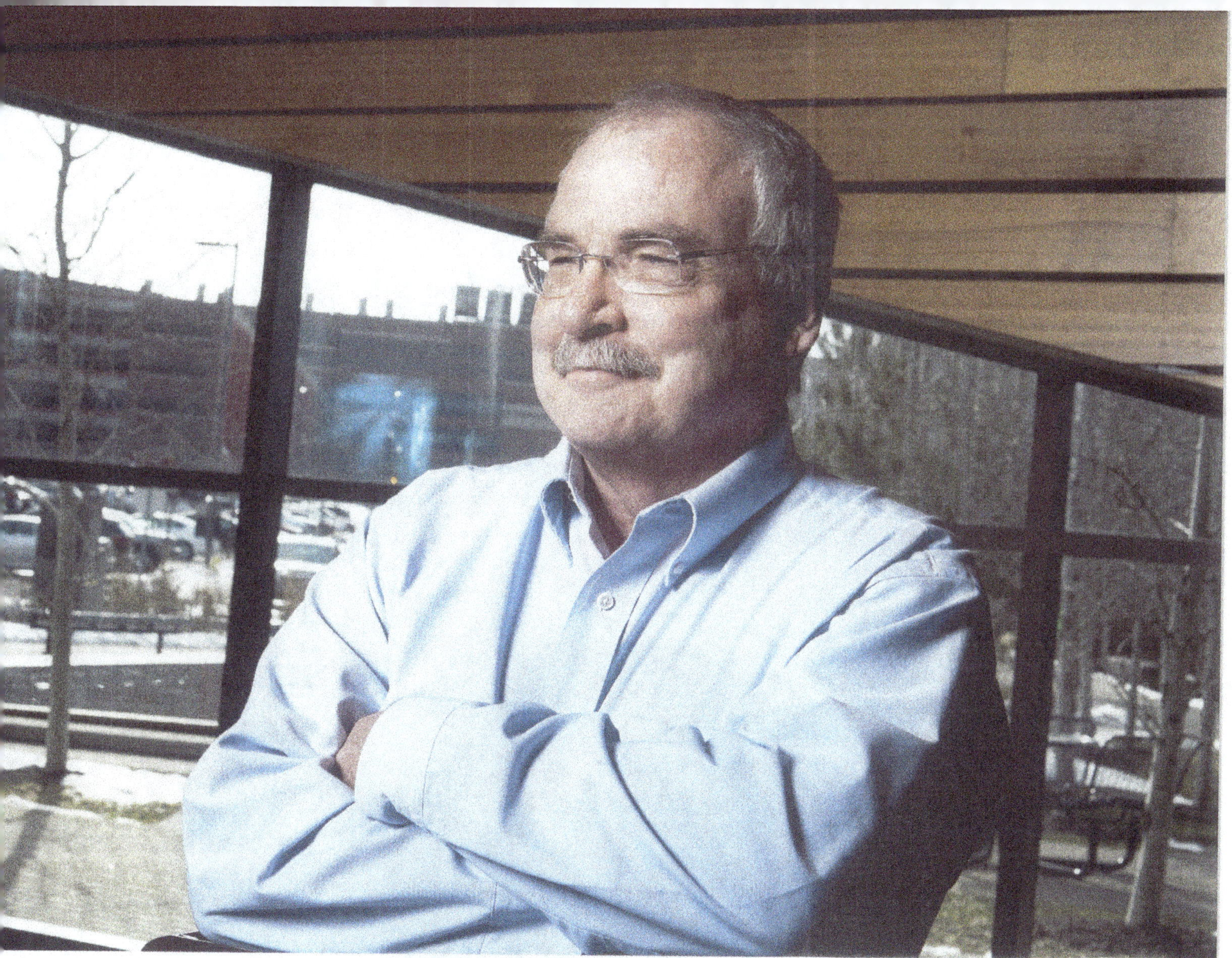

ALL POSSIBILITIES

Just after Glenn hired me, we were walking along, and he said, "If you make decisions that I don't agree with, I will give you the chance to convince me. If you convince me, then I will support you. If I'm not convinced, I will still support you."

I remember that walk and his confidence in me. And it's been 27 years.

LEN WEISS
DIRECTOR OF THE APOLLO CENTER

Glenn is an extremely creative, fly-by-the-seat-of-his-pants guy. He was gung-ho to do anything that he thought would help clients. In fact, sometimes you'd have to say, "Glenn, I don't think we can pull that off."

MARY KAY MCJILTON
VICE PRESIDENT

FIGHT STIGMA
Wear a T-Shirt

Get one of these shirts from your favorite
online store—or create your own!
What's your personal mental health message?

*Mental illness is nothing to
be ashamed of, but stigma
and bias shame us all.*
— BILL CLINTON

*Could you love
someone with
mental illness?
You probably do.*

¡UST BREATHE
*(If you don't know the significance
of the semicolon, check out Page 46!)*

**THE MORE YOU KNOW
THE LESS YOU JUDGE
Mental Illness
Awareness**

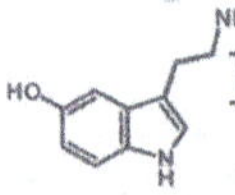

*Depression
is a flaw in*
CHEMISTRY,
not
CHARACTER

#IMNOTASHAMED

*no one can
stigmatize me
without my
permission*

**I HAVE A
MENTAL ILLNESS
Let's Talk
About It**

**IT'S OK
NOT TO BE OK**

**I am anxious
I am depressed
I AM HUMAN**

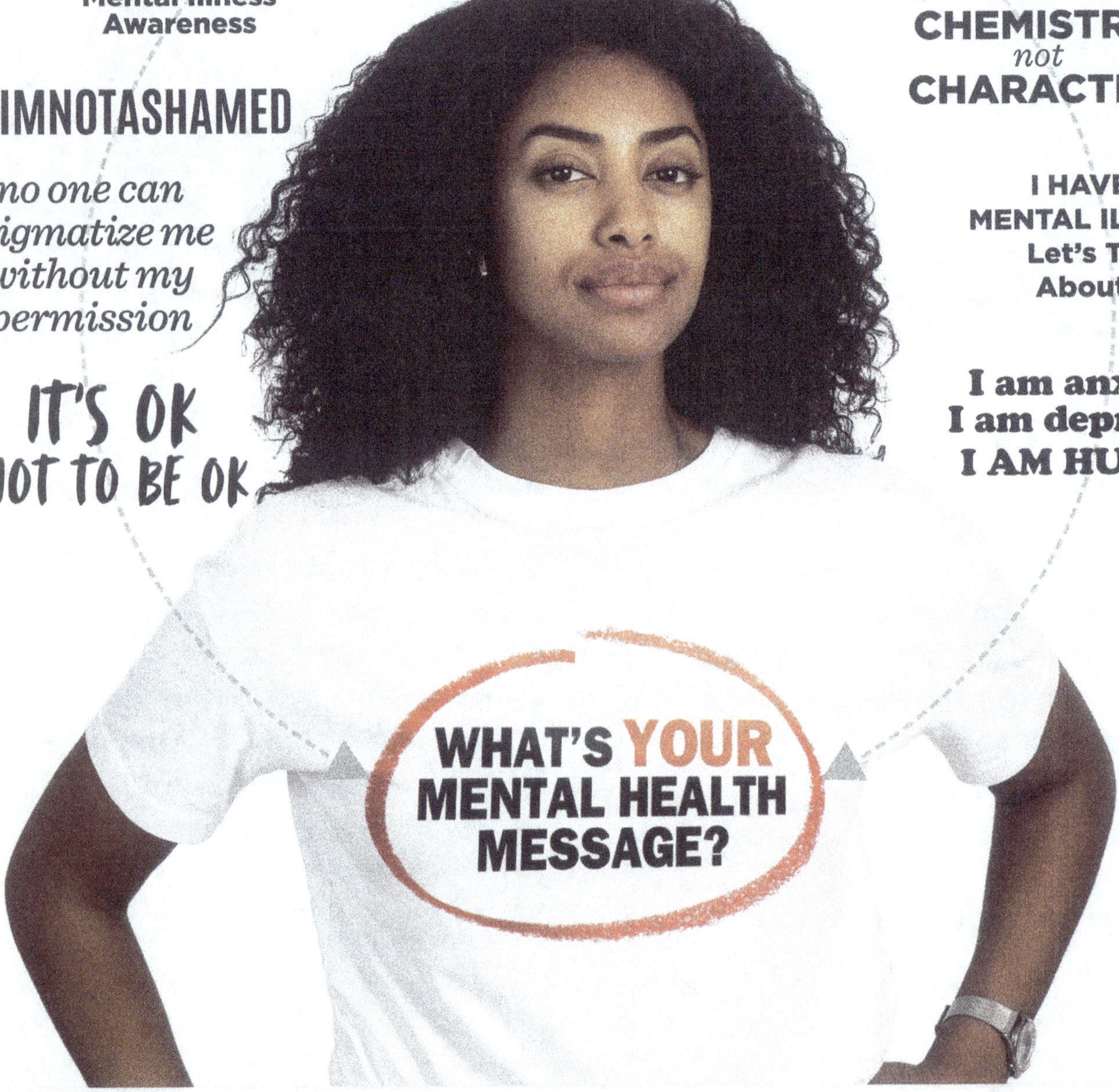

**WHAT'S YOUR
MENTAL HEALTH
MESSAGE?**

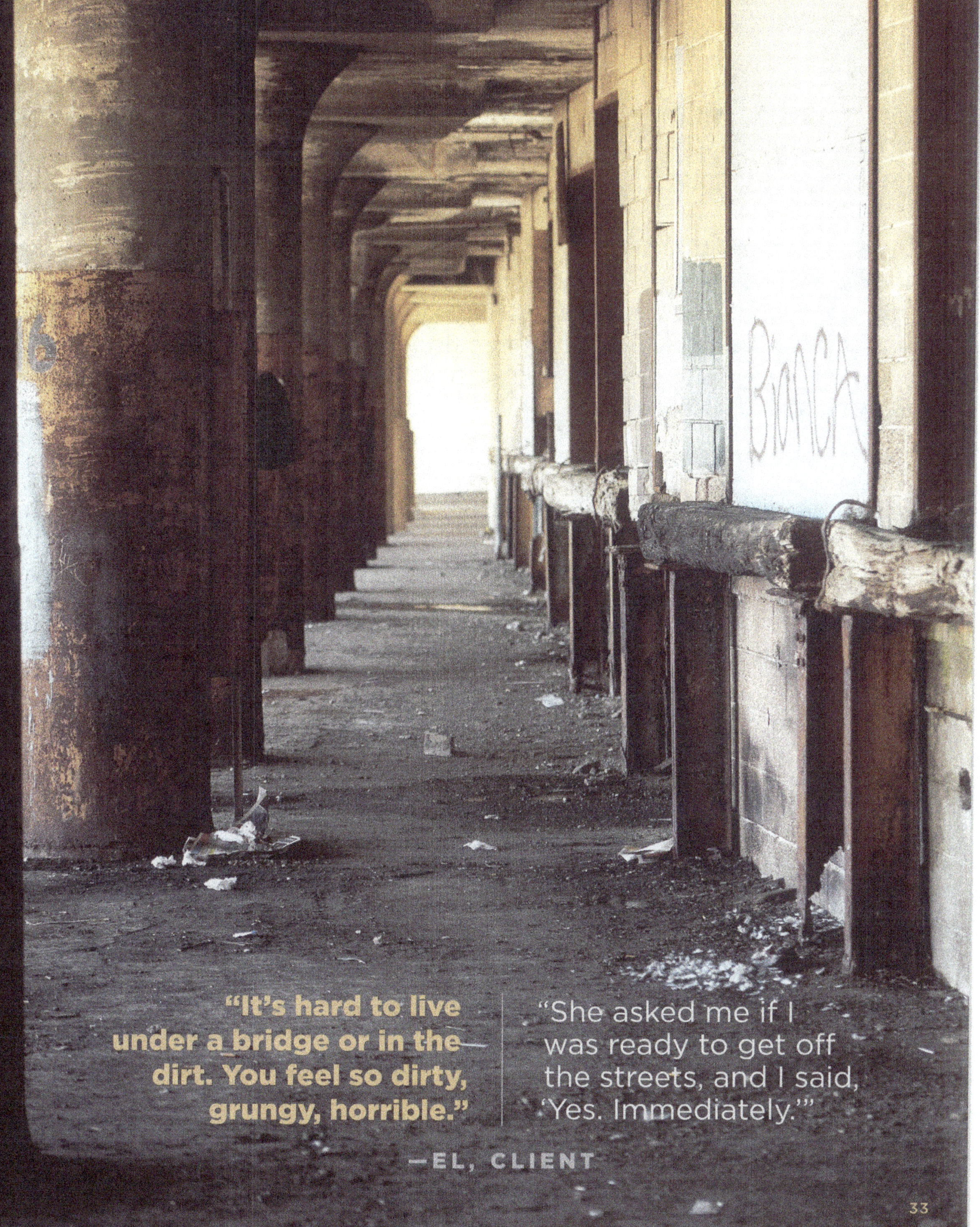
"It's hard to live under a bridge or in the dirt. You feel so dirty, grungy, horrible."

"She asked me if I was ready to get off the streets, and I said, 'Yes. Immediately.'"

—EL, CLIENT

BACK IN THE DAY, if you were homeless and had a mental illness, you just—hung out there. You went into a shelter, then maybe you went back to the street, you went to a flop-house to live for a while, you got put into jail, you went back onto the street...

—TIM BURKETT, FORMER CEO

Imagine trying to keep track of your meds, reconnect with your family, or make one more attempt to stay sober—when you don't even know where you're sleeping tonight.

In 2004, we started our Safe Haven programs. People with mental illness could move from the streets into one of our stable homes with access to the treatment they needed.

Today, we're still helping people find transitional housing. And when they feel ready, they can move into permanent housing with supportive services.

"I used to sleep with a hammer in case someone tried to attack me in the middle of the night."

"I was so shocked that a program like this even existed. It's so different than the shelters and the usual approach."

—BRIAN, CLIENT

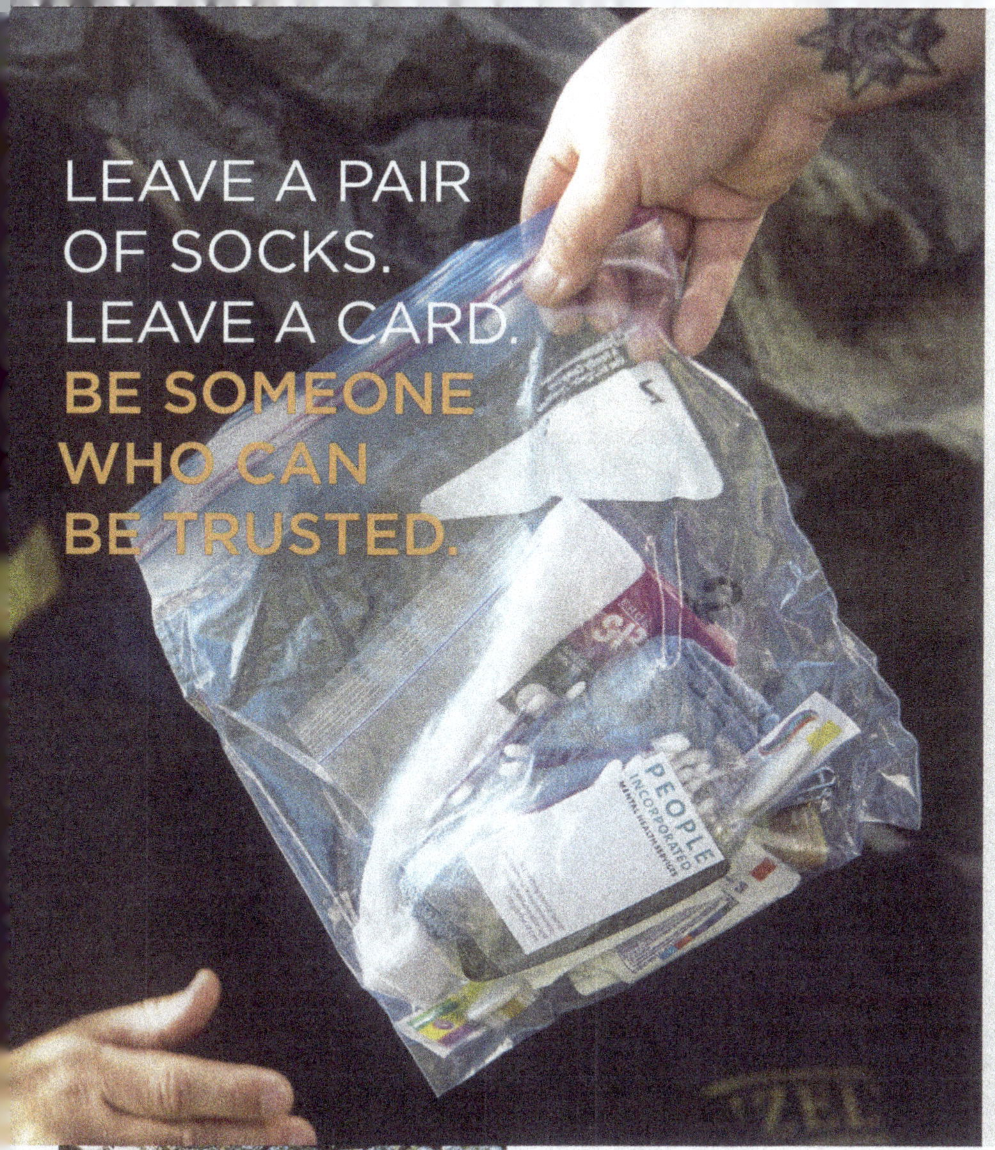

LEAVE A PAIR
OF SOCKS.
LEAVE A CARD.
BE SOMEONE
WHO CAN
BE TRUSTED.

The homeless
outreach that People
Incorporated does
is really effective.
Those workers really
know how to engage
people to develop
trust and get them into
treatment and housing.

—Sue Abderholden
 NAMI-MN

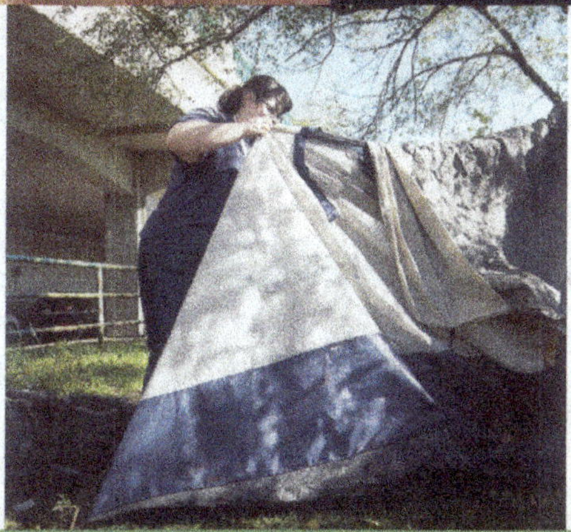

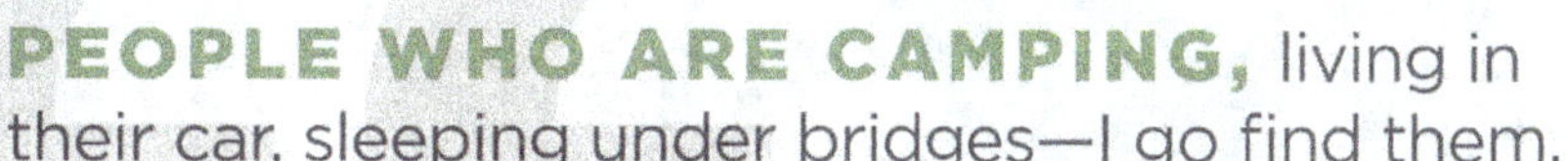

PEOPLE WHO ARE CAMPING, living in
their car, sleeping under bridges—I go find them.

—ALYSSA, OUTREACH WORKER

"I just wanted to get out of it.
To figure out how to get
my life back."

"They had an **OPEN** door
and an **OPEN** ear."

—WILLIE, CLIENT

OPEN TO WHATEVER

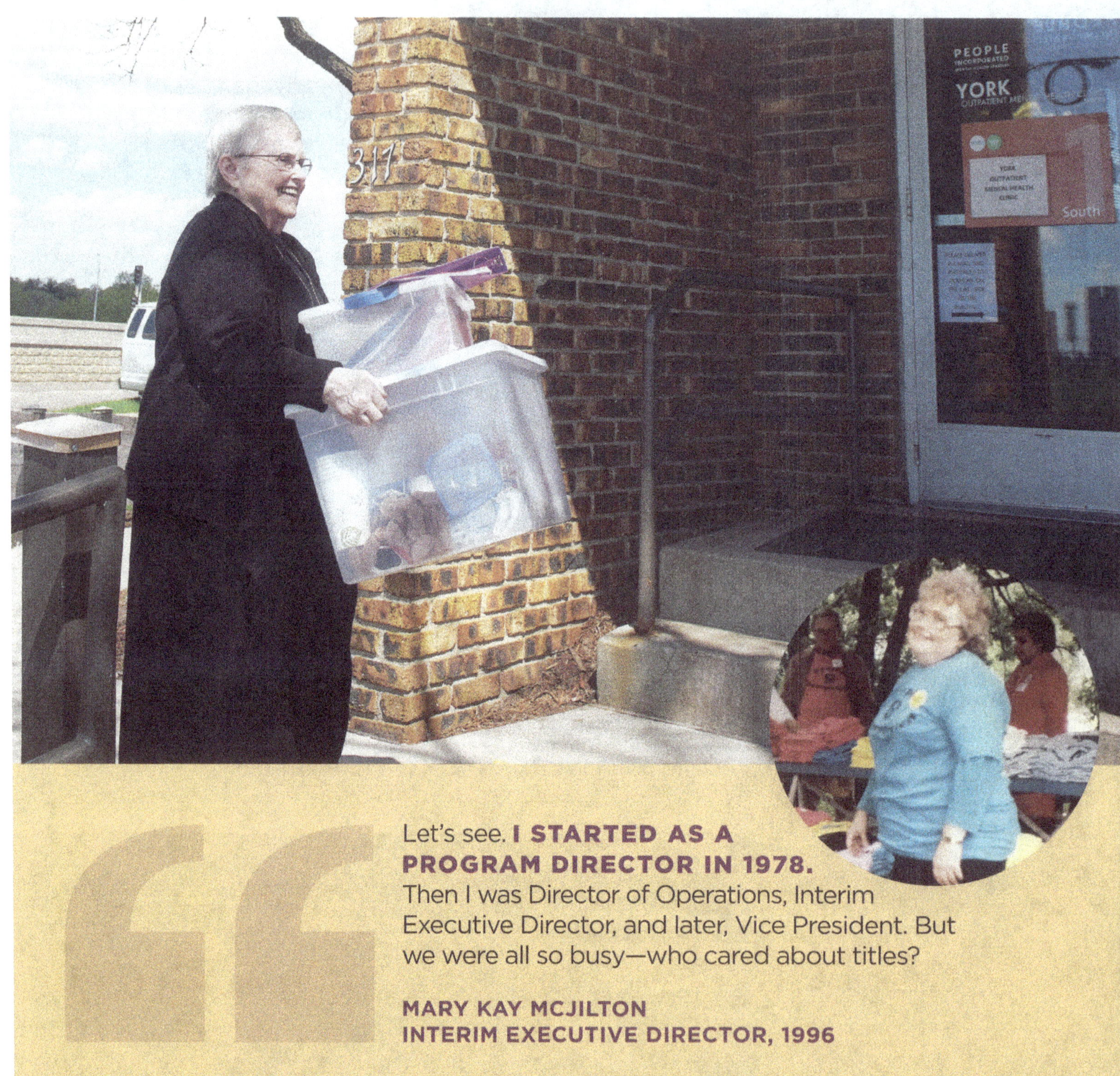

Let's see. **I STARTED AS A PROGRAM DIRECTOR IN 1978.** Then I was Director of Operations, Interim Executive Director, and later, Vice President. But we were all so busy—who cared about titles?

MARY KAY MCJILTON
INTERIM EXECUTIVE DIRECTOR, 1996

NEEDED DOING

An excerpt from an interview with Mary Kay

INTERVIEWER: *You were the Interim Executive Director for just under six months?*

MARY KAY: Right. They needed somebody to fill in between Glenn (Anderson) and Tim (Burkett).

INTERVIEWER: *But for the 18 years before that, and another 15 years after, until you retired, you were pretty integral to the running of the place.*

MARY KAY: I guess I was the Can-Do Person. Bring me a problem, and I'll figure it out. You need a proposal? I'll write it. You need flowers planted? Diapers washed at Children's Services? Okay.

INTERVIEWER: *What were the early days like for you?*

MARY KAY: We were growing so fast, it started to become overwhelming. There wasn't enough of an infrastructure. You felt like you were putting your finger in the dyke in about six different places all the time.

" MARY KAY WAS A MIRACLE WORKER.

**LANCE HOLTHUSEN
PEER SUPPORT SPECIALIST**

INTERVIEWER: *You've known this organization so intimately, for so long. Where does it shine?*

MARY KAY: We take on challenges. We try things that aren't being done in the community. Also, the staff, the leadership, and the board really care about each individual. We always see a client as a whole person—who maybe has a mental health issue.

AUTHOR'S NOTE: *Mary Kay retired in 2011 when her husband became ill. She volunteered for a couple of years and came back on staff in 2013 as an Administrative Assistant. As she puts it:*

"I'll keep working here as long as they'll have me—and I don't screw anything up."

Mary Kay was my boss most of the time. And I say, to this day, she's the best boss I ever had.

JOAN, PROGRAM DIRECTOR

Mary Kay was very, very beloved. Very, very generous. She never gave up on anybody.

TIM BURKETT, FORMER CEO

You talk about a walking People Incorporated person! Mary Kay McJilton was inspirational. She put her heart and soul into making a difference for all the people we served.

BARBARA NICHOLS, VICE PRESIDENT OF COMMUNITY RELATIONS

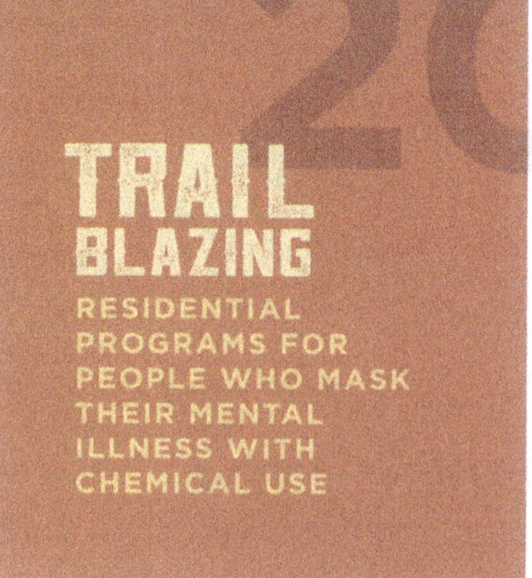

Great American Cowboys

Fighting for People with Co-Occurring Diagnoses

A cowboy can hear a hawk change direction on the wind a mile away but can't seem to hear the word *impossible*.

When a person with mental illness wants to break free of their chemical dependency, the dual-diagnosis can make it doubly hard.

So the People Incorporated Cowboys blazed a new trail to help ease their way.

From TIM, DIRECTOR OF QUALITY ASSURANCE:
In the traditional addiction community, there's a split. You have to do the alcohol and chemical dependency treatment first, before you can treat the mental illness.

From TIM BURKETT, FORMER CEO:
If you're not abstinent, you're out of here, basically. And that requirement hadn't been working very well for people self-medicating for mental illness.

UPDATE!
This approach, which began as our grand experiment, is now common practice in Minnesota.

So in spite of strong cautions from chemical dependency experts, Tim Burkett spearheaded bringing a co-occurring model here from California. In other words, we now treat both mental illness and chemical dependency at the same time.

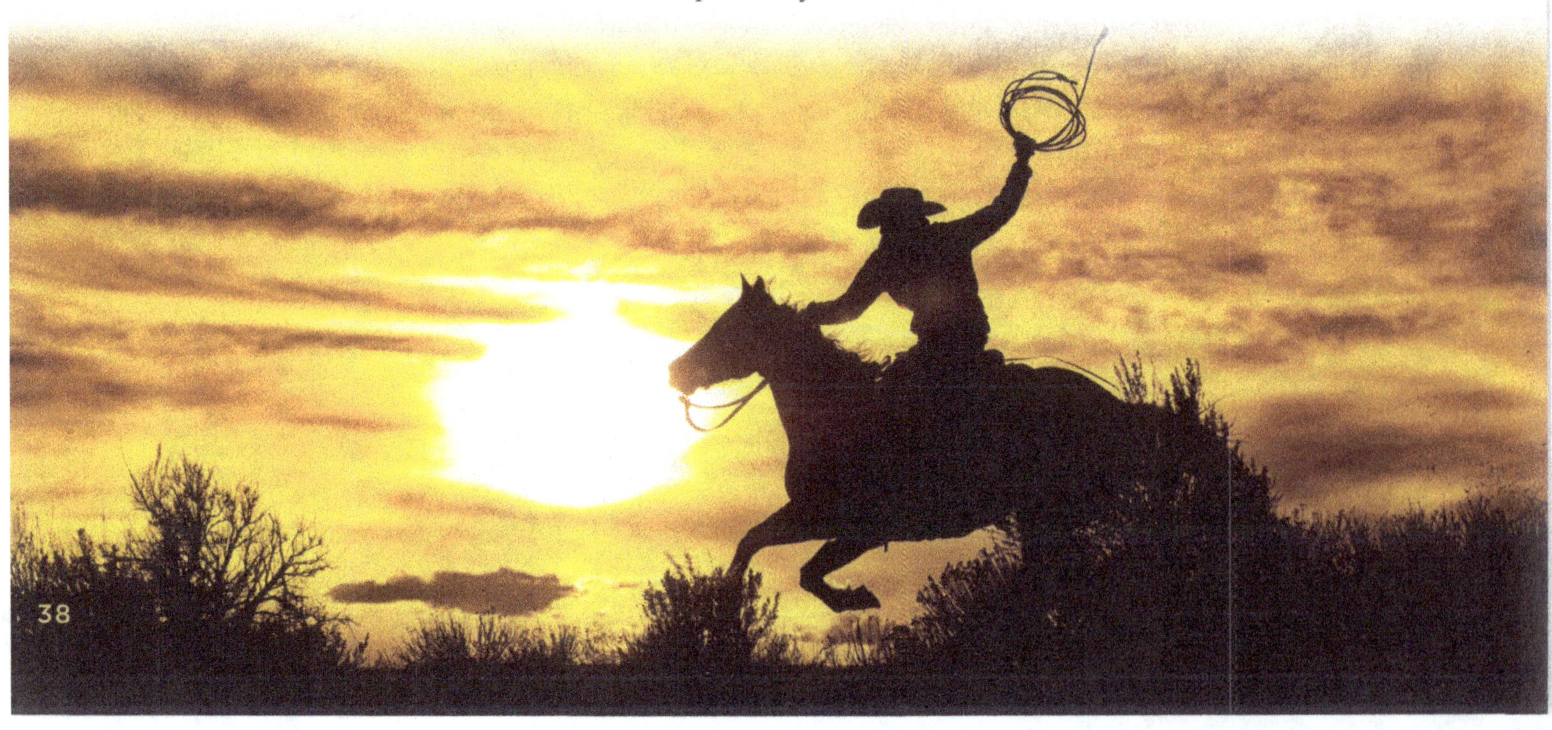

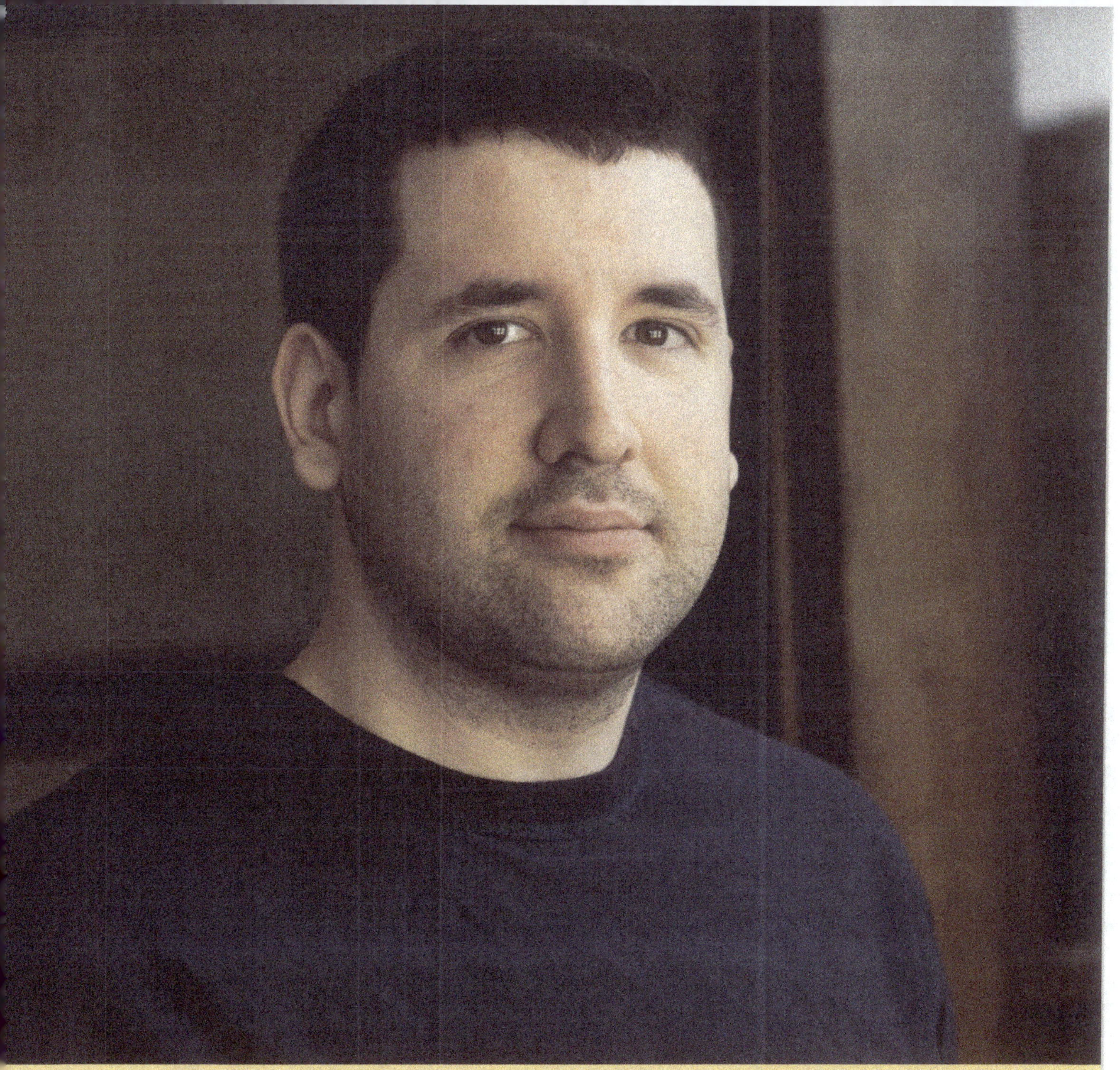

MEET KYLE.

He hardly left his house for 3 years.

Today he goes out running and wins paintball awards.

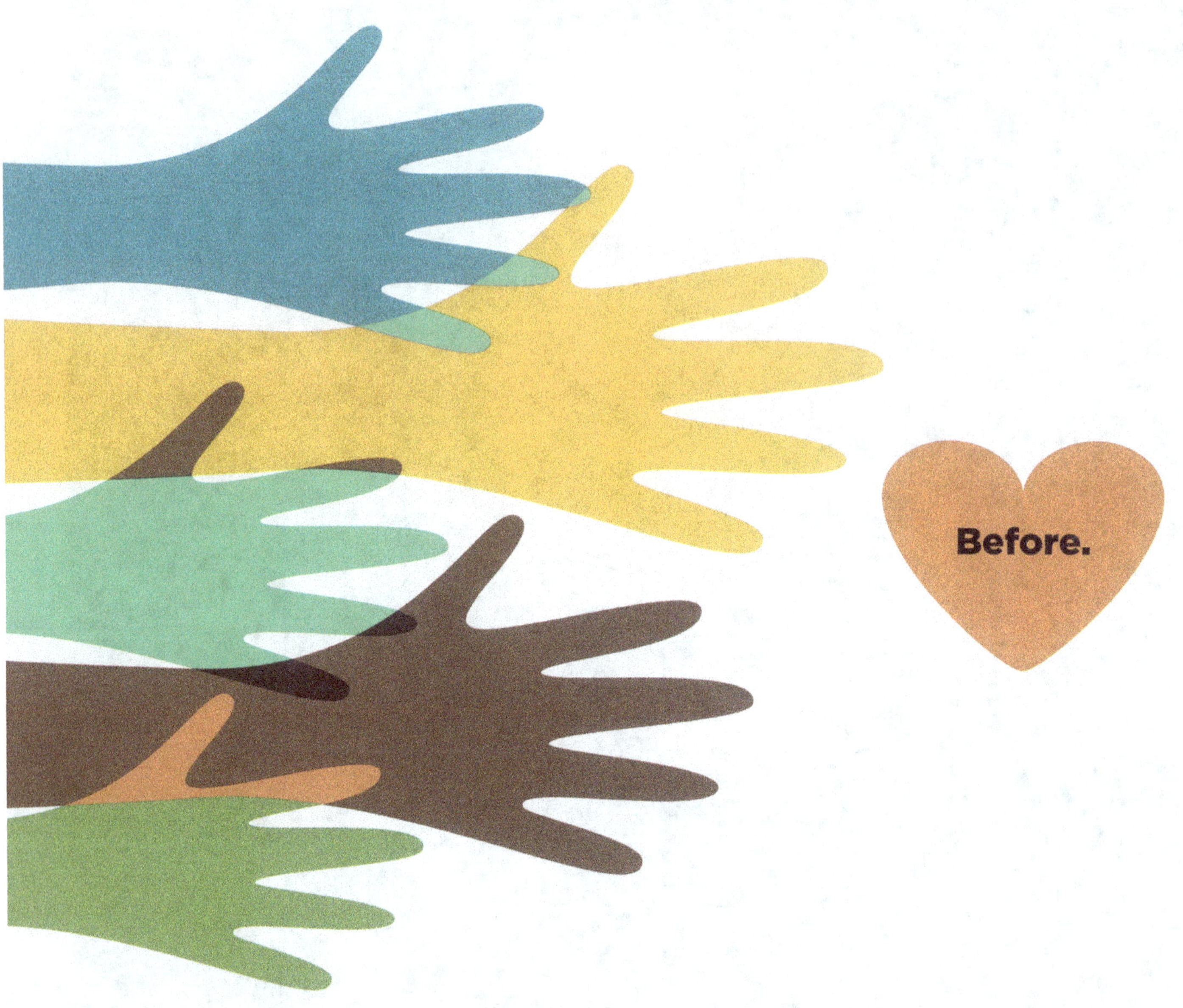

We're Evolving

We've spent most of the past half-century developing 40+ individual programs to care for people with mental illness.

Pardon our brag, but this means every client has had access to a range of remarkable services and a staff of people standing by to help.

That said, a client who is cared for by lots of unconnected programs can spend more time trying to find resources than getting their needs met. And we're sorry about that.

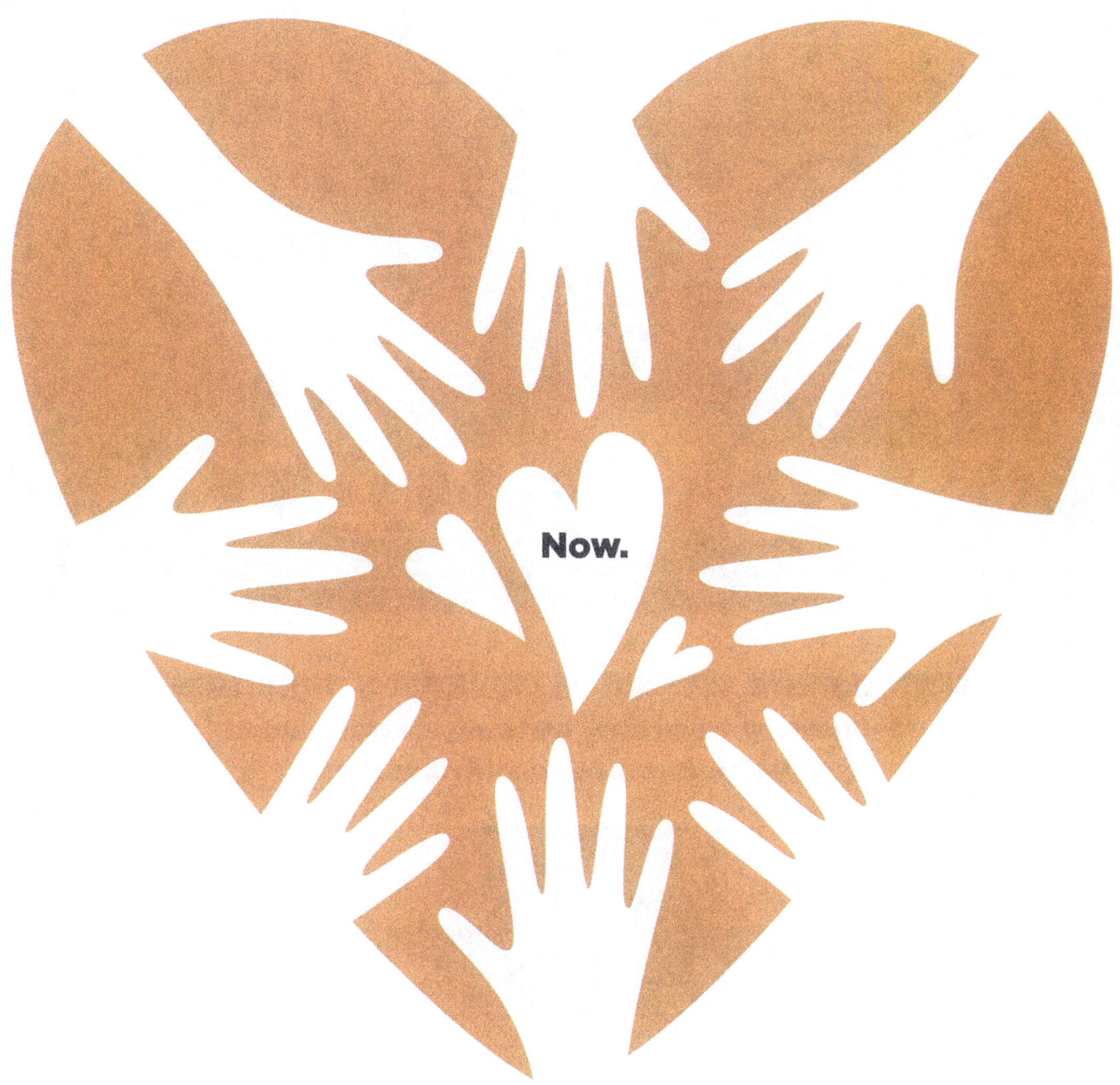

Today we're surrounding each client with a single unified system of care.

One **WHOLE PERSON** on the road to recovery. One goal plan. One solid commitment to being there.

Life is dynamic. A person may need very different services next year than this year. And now we're in a better position to help the most vulnerable among us reach their full potential.

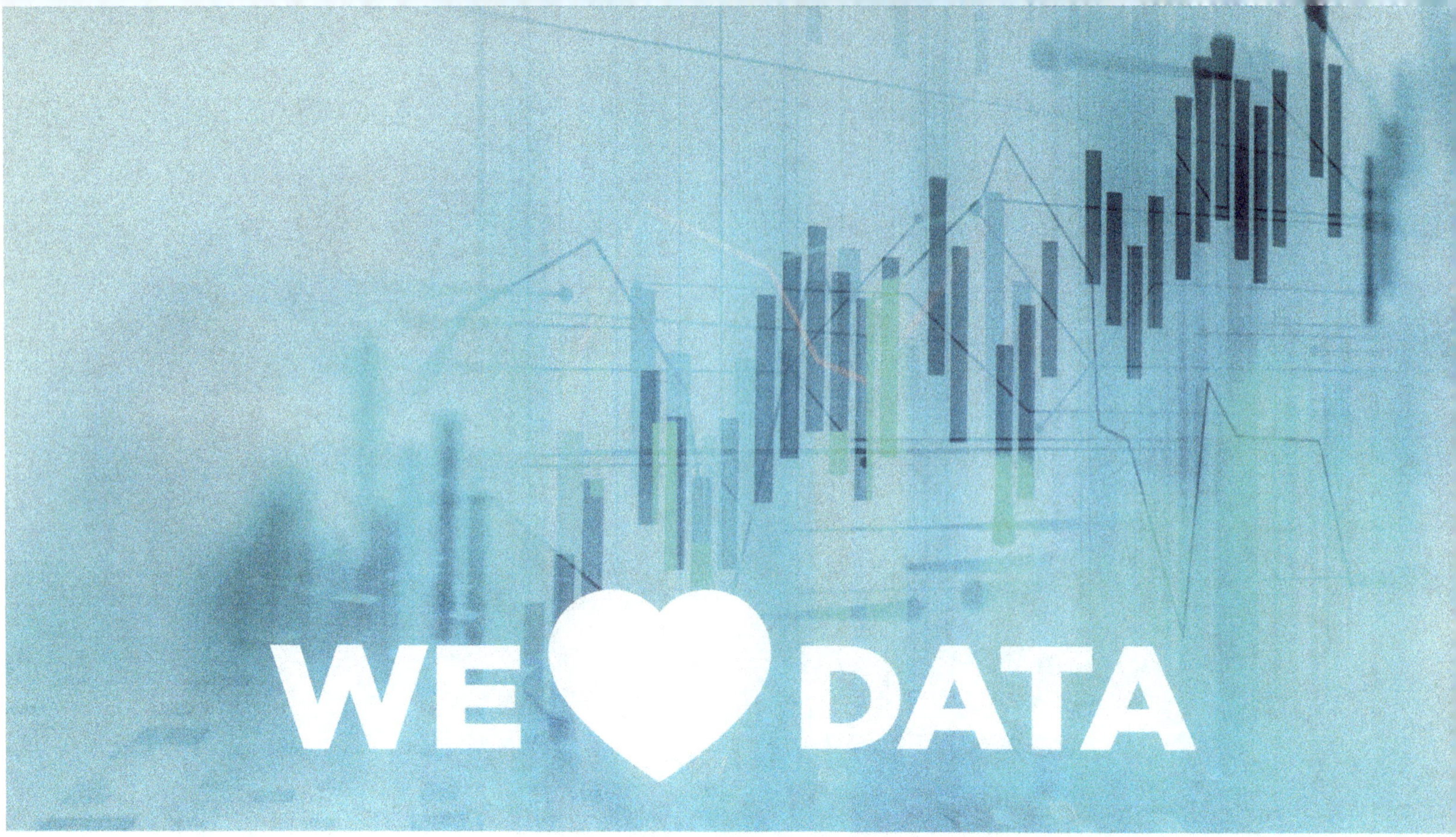

WE ♥ DATA

AROUND HERE, WE'RE BIG BELIEVERS IN EVIDENCE.

We're not satisfied until we track, measure, survey, analyze, re-measure, and re-analyze.

We made a difference for our CLIENTS

81%
felt their condition had somewhat or greatly improved

77%
said they could deal more effectively with daily problems

We made a difference for our COMMUNITY

Treating our clients for crisis-related depression cost

3.5 million dollars less

than it would have cost at a hospital

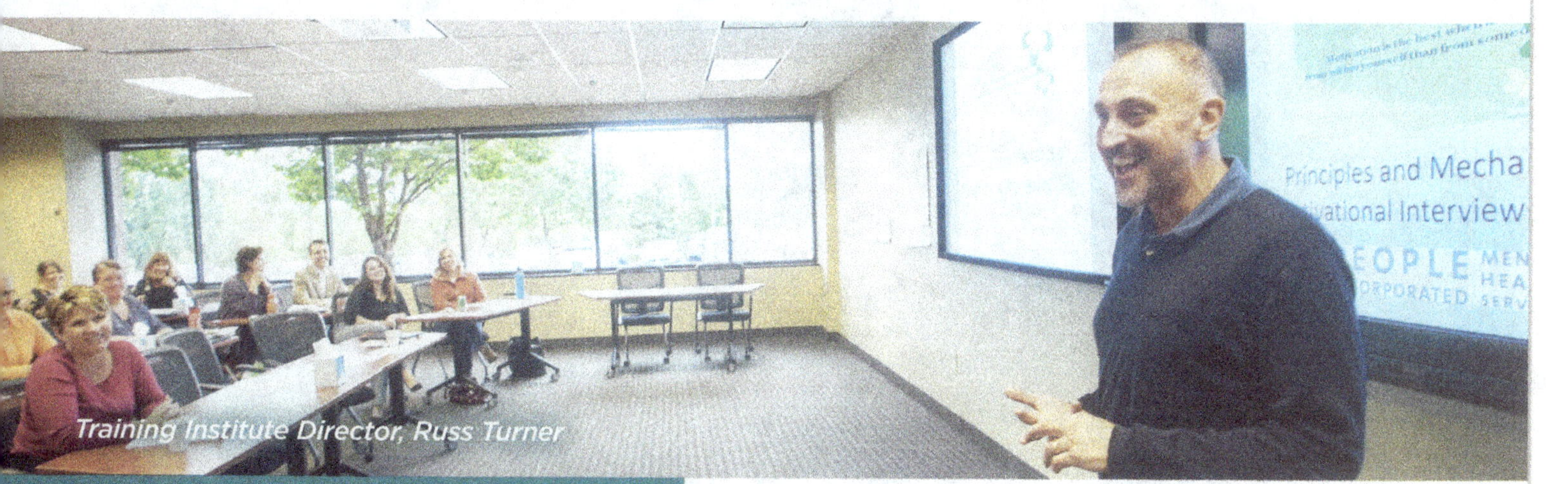

Training Institute Director, Russ Turner

Our Training Institute offers classes to our own staff, other health professionals in the field, and anyone who wants to learn more about mental health.

Part of the reason for creating the institute was to establish the organization as a place like the Mayo Clinic—where the entire community could benefit from the expertise.

JAN ANDERSON, FORMER BOARD CHAIR

I've worked at places that do no training at all. They say, "Here's the key to your office—now go help homeless people." But here they say, "You need to take all of these classes so you know how to help our clients."

KATIE, OUTREACH CASE MANAGER

I've done some training through the institute. I want the staff to know that even the sickest people they deal with have the ability to get better. We can go on to live really wonderful lives.

MELANIE, CLIENT

SHARING KNOWLEDGE WITH THE COMMUNITY

One of our Licensed Social Workers, Amber Ruth, is embedded with the St. Paul Police Department. This collaboration helps officers make more informed and person-centered decisions on crisis calls involving people with mental illness.

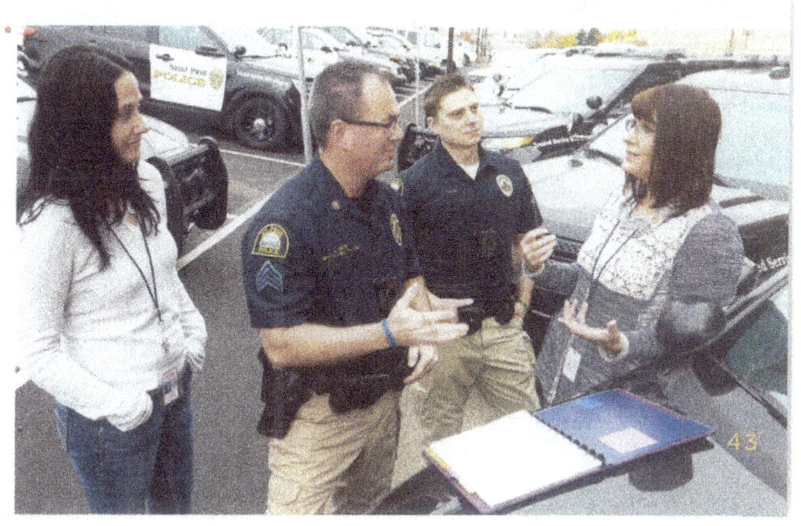

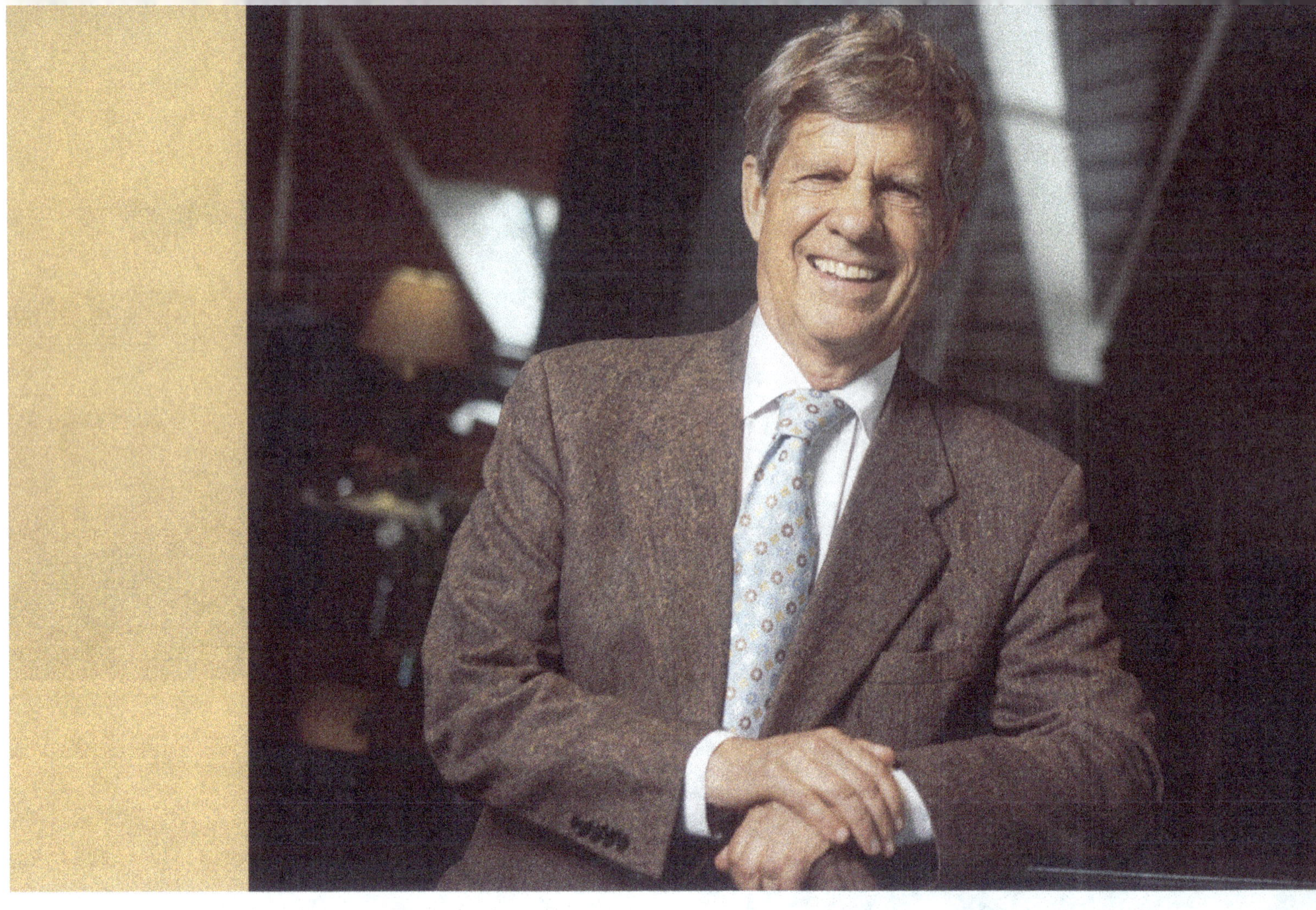

OPEN TO SHAKING

An excerpt from an interview with Tim

INTERVIEWER: *What made you want to join the People Incorporated ranks?*

TIM: They were doing all kinds of experimental programs for people with deafness and mental illness, for women with mental illness, for people with seizure disorders and mental illness. They had moved in where angels feared to tread.

INTERVIEWER: *And what was your overarching philosophy during your tenure?*

TIM: I wanted to bring this condition into the mainstream, so that people with mental illness could get the respect they needed to feel like real citizens who could offer something to this community.

INTERVIEWER: *Along with creating new programs, you worked to change the organization's public image, yes?*

TIM: I bought a whole wardrobe of suits. I wore one every day. We were going to become part of the establishment, damn it! We were going to attract the movers and shakers, and they were going to move and shake with us, and our clients were going to feel accepted and supported. And it happened!

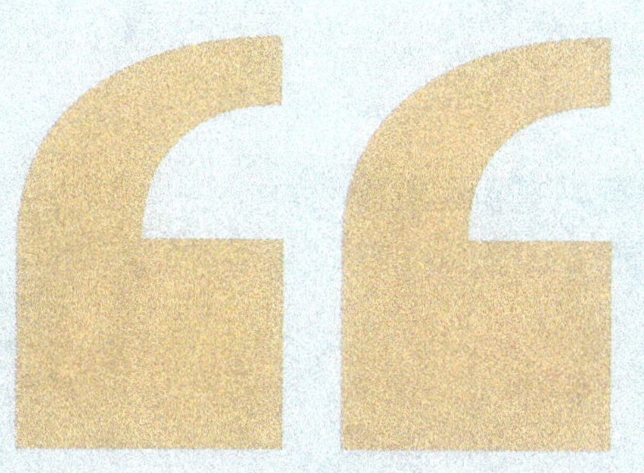

WHAT I KNEW ABOUT PEOPLE INCORPORATED WAS THAT THEY WERE A JEWEL IN THE ROUGH THAT NOBODY HAD HEARD ABOUT.

They were the only organization who would take on this demeaned group of people as legitimate citizens. And they had a founder who sounded pretty cool.

—TIM BURKETT, FORMER CEO, 1996-2014

HE JUST BELIEVED, I THINK, AT HIS MOST CORE LEVEL, THAT THERE WAS HOPE FOR EVERY SINGLE INDIVIDUAL. BUT SOCIETY HAD EXCLUDED THESE INDIVIDUALS FROM THAT COMMON CONVERSATION. AND HE WAS NOT GOING TO LET THAT HAPPEN.

JILL WIEDEMANN-WEST, CEO

Tim drew good people because he was good people. He became a very effective CEO, even though he was a social worker at heart. And he was——is *brilliant* too strong a term?

ALDEN DREW
FORMER BOARD MEMBER

THINGS UP

During my watch, this place grew, maybe, threefold. But Tim Burkett took it off like a rocket after I left. He's a Zen Buddhist. And I think he was always at a quiet place and very thoughtful and strategic.

GLENN ANDERSON, FORMER EXECUTIVE DIRECTOR

Well I think Tim never saw an opportunity that we should not go after. That was definitely his philosophy.

MARY KAY MCJILTON, VICE PRESIDENT

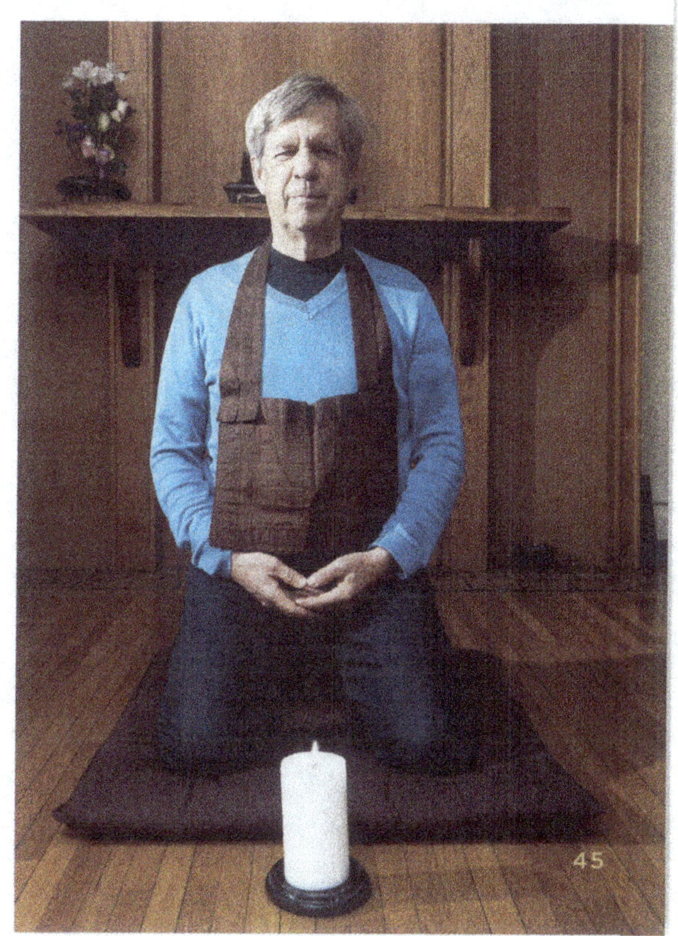

Tim is now the Guiding Teacher at the Minnesota Zen Meditation Center

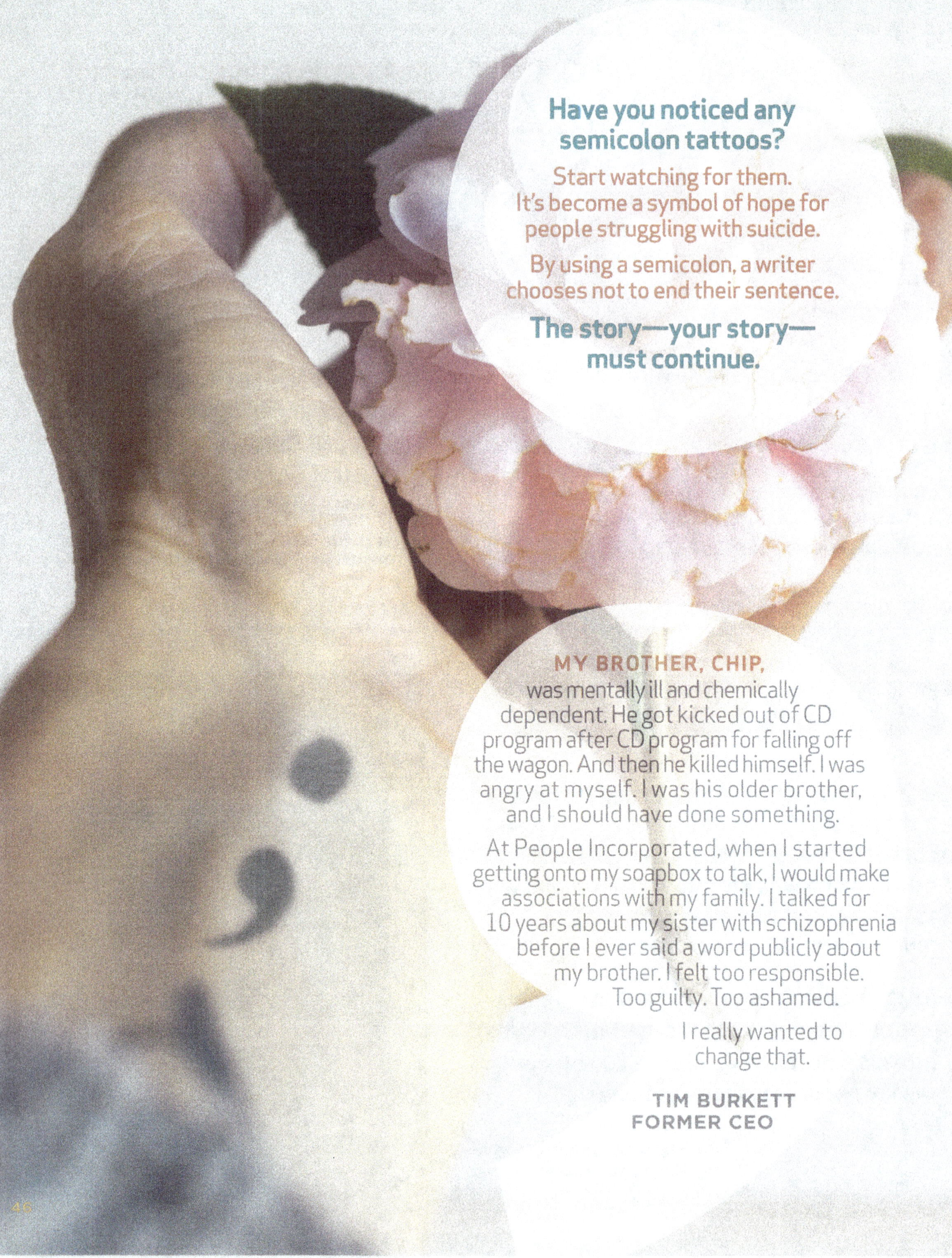

Have you noticed any semicolon tattoos?

Start watching for them. It's become a symbol of hope for people struggling with suicide.

By using a semicolon, a writer chooses not to end their sentence.

The story—your story—must continue.

MY BROTHER, CHIP, was mentally ill and chemically dependent. He got kicked out of CD program after CD program for falling off the wagon. And then he killed himself. I was angry at myself. I was his older brother, and I should have done something.

At People Incorporated, when I started getting onto my soapbox to talk, I would make associations with my family. I talked for 10 years about my sister with schizophrenia before I ever said a word publicly about my brother. I felt too responsible. Too guilty. Too ashamed.

I really wanted to change that.

TIM BURKETT
FORMER CEO

From TIM BURKETT, FORMER CEO:

This radical idea was that you don't lock these people up. You create a home for them for several days while they're in crisis. And then you help them move on. Everyone warned us: "Don't do this!" But we went ahead. And now it's the new normal.

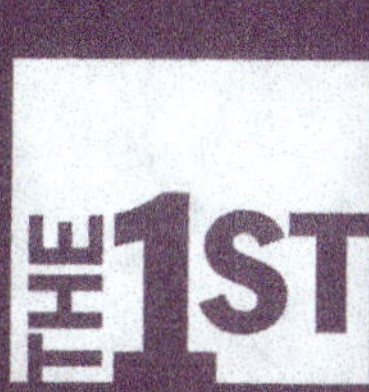

THE FIRST CRISIS RESIDENCE IN MINNESOTA FOR PEOPLE WITH MENTAL ILLNESS

Great American Cowboys

Fighting for Crisis Residences

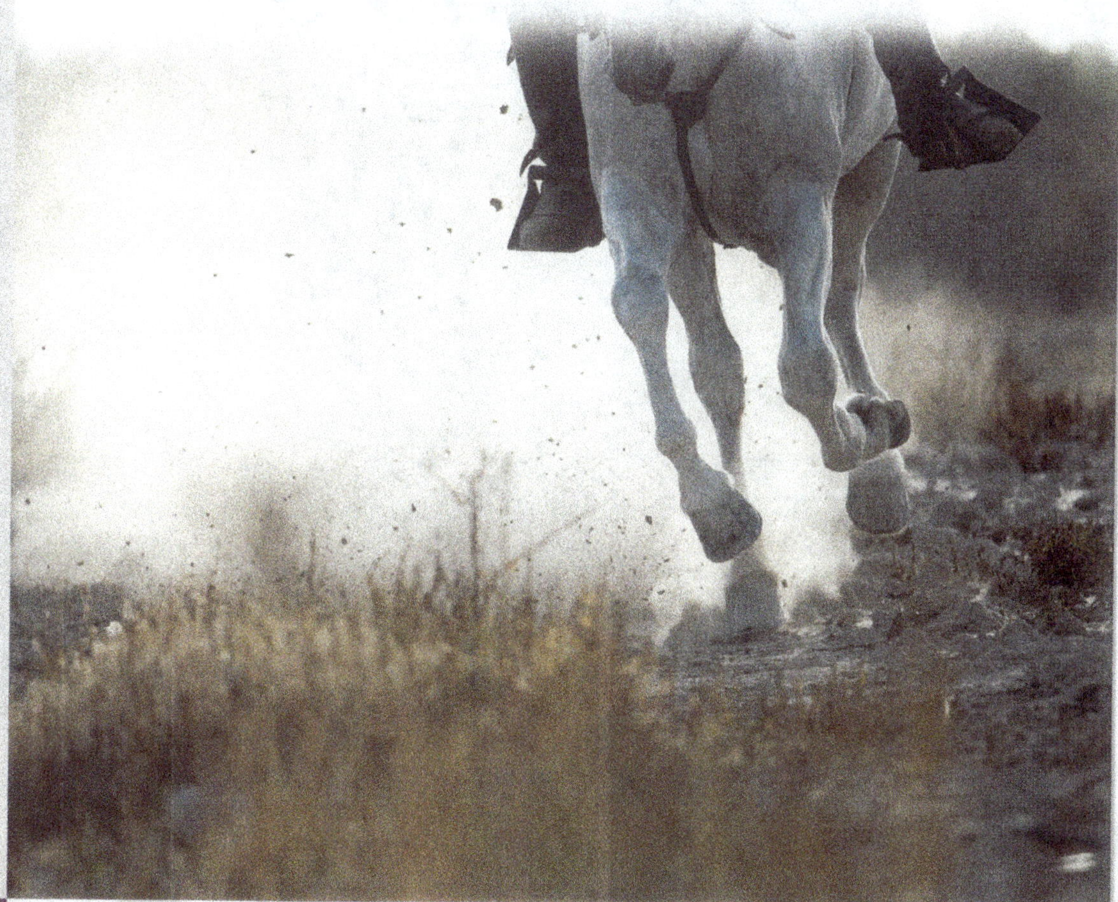

From KATHRYN, SENIOR PROGRAM MANAGER:

It's an honor to sit with somebody and hear the story of all that they've come through. And yet here they are, poking their head up, trying to shine again—even though it's been raining so hard.

From JAN ANDERSON, FORMER BOARD CHAIR:

My daughter was served in the People Incorporated crisis centers a couple of times. And she confessed that she acted out, in the hopes that she could stay a little longer.

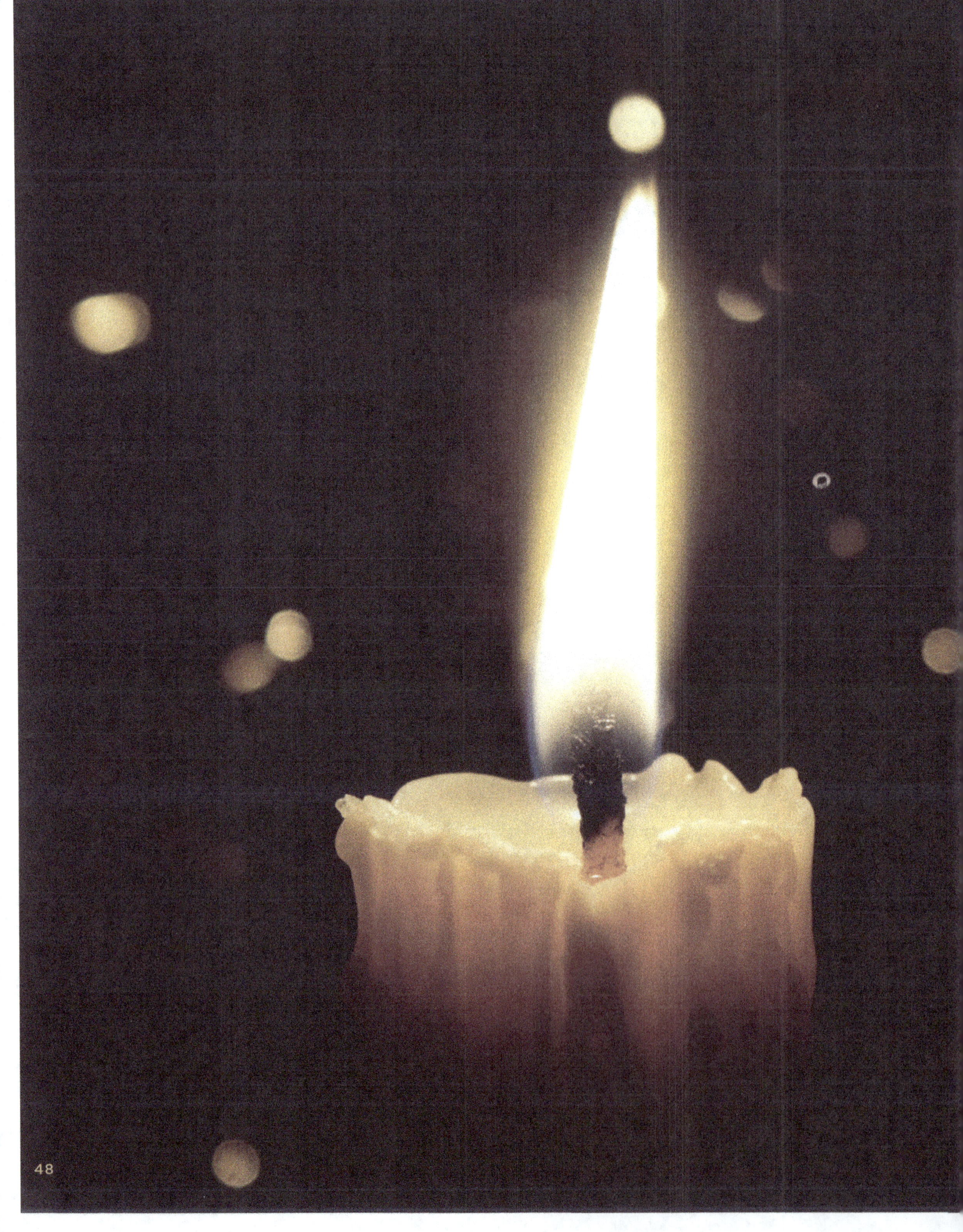

Allow yourself a moment of
doubt when the media reports
that mental illness is behind a
violent tragedy.

People with mental illness are
far more likely to be victims of
violence than to commit violence.

THE PEOPLE WHO PEOPLE

A mental health crisis can unravel a person's functioning. But we don't lose hope. When our client has lost their hope, we hold it for them until they're ready to pick it up again.

KATHRYN, SENIOR PROGRAM MANAGER

PEOPLE INCORPORATED STAFF FILL KINDESS KITS FOR THE HOMELESS. NOT BECAUSE THEY'RE ASKED TO, BUT BECAUSE THEY ASK TO.

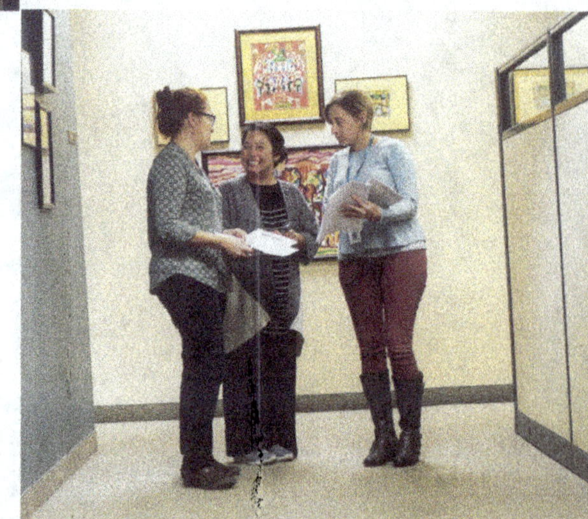

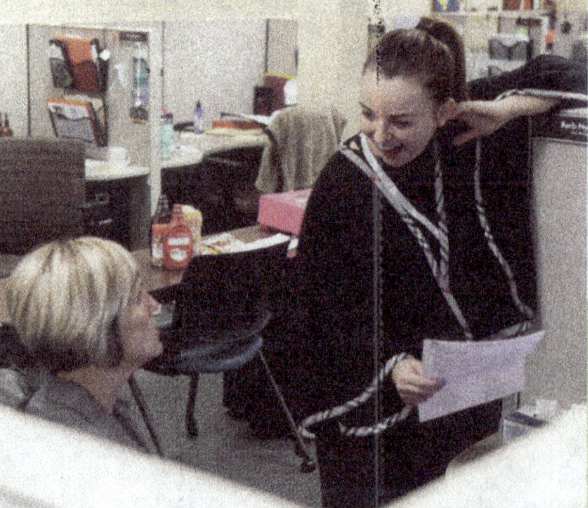

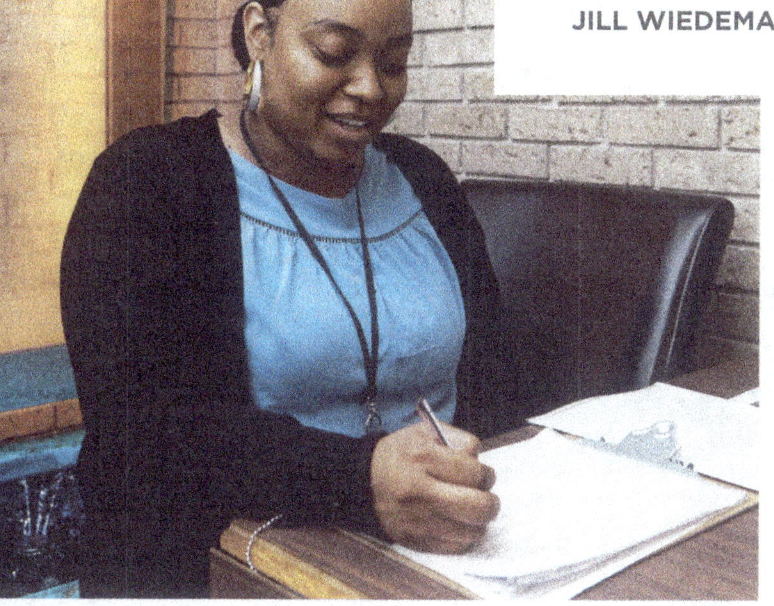

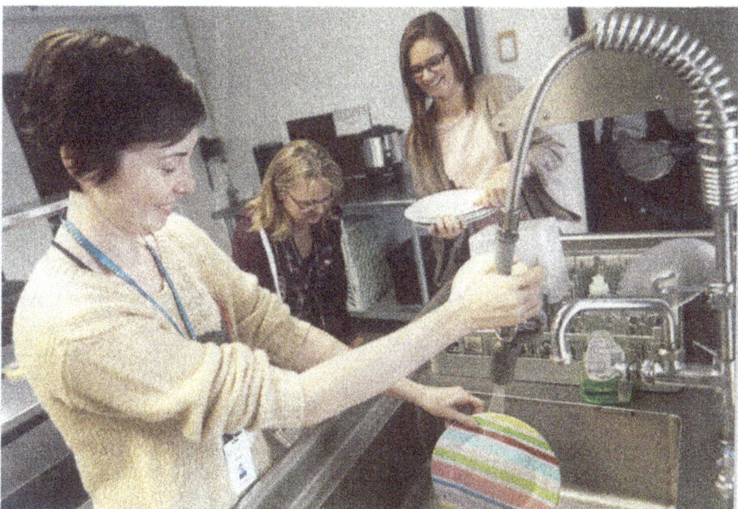

PEOPLE INCORPORATED

I was working outside, and one of the clients came up and just started talking about what he'd been going through and what his addictions were. More than anything, I just listened. At the end of the conversation I just said to him, "Well, you know what? You're in a safe environment. You're in the right place to get the help you need."

He was a big dude. He grabbed me and gave me a bear hug and said, "Amen, Brother!" Then he just turned and walked away.

JOE, FACILITIES

People would always ask me, "Why do you continue to work there? Because it sounds pretty desperate at times." And I'd always say, "Because people there really care."
MARY KAY MCJILTON, VICE PRESIDENT

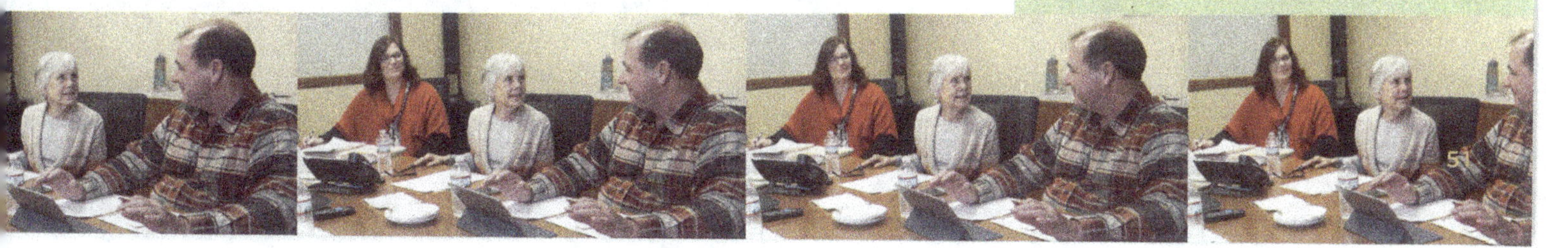

I HAVE AUDITORY HALLUCINATIONS.
I HEAR 38 DIFFERENT VOICES.

And I actually hear them as I talk to you. They all have a different tone pitch, so they all have names. My voices are totally negative. All of them. Trying to kill me. Wanting me dead. Not good enough to live.

I wanted to be well. I've wanted it so bad I could taste it. I did give up for awhile. I was three times suicide. You're always being beaten down by these voices.

I was homeless, and my son took me in. His wife was just having a baby. And he didn't want to see me in the street anymore. I shared the room with the baby. I loved it. My granddaughter brought hope back to me. It was the *being born again* piece. 'Cause I started remembering what my life was like before I heard the voices. Just free-running and everything. And I wanted to capture that again.

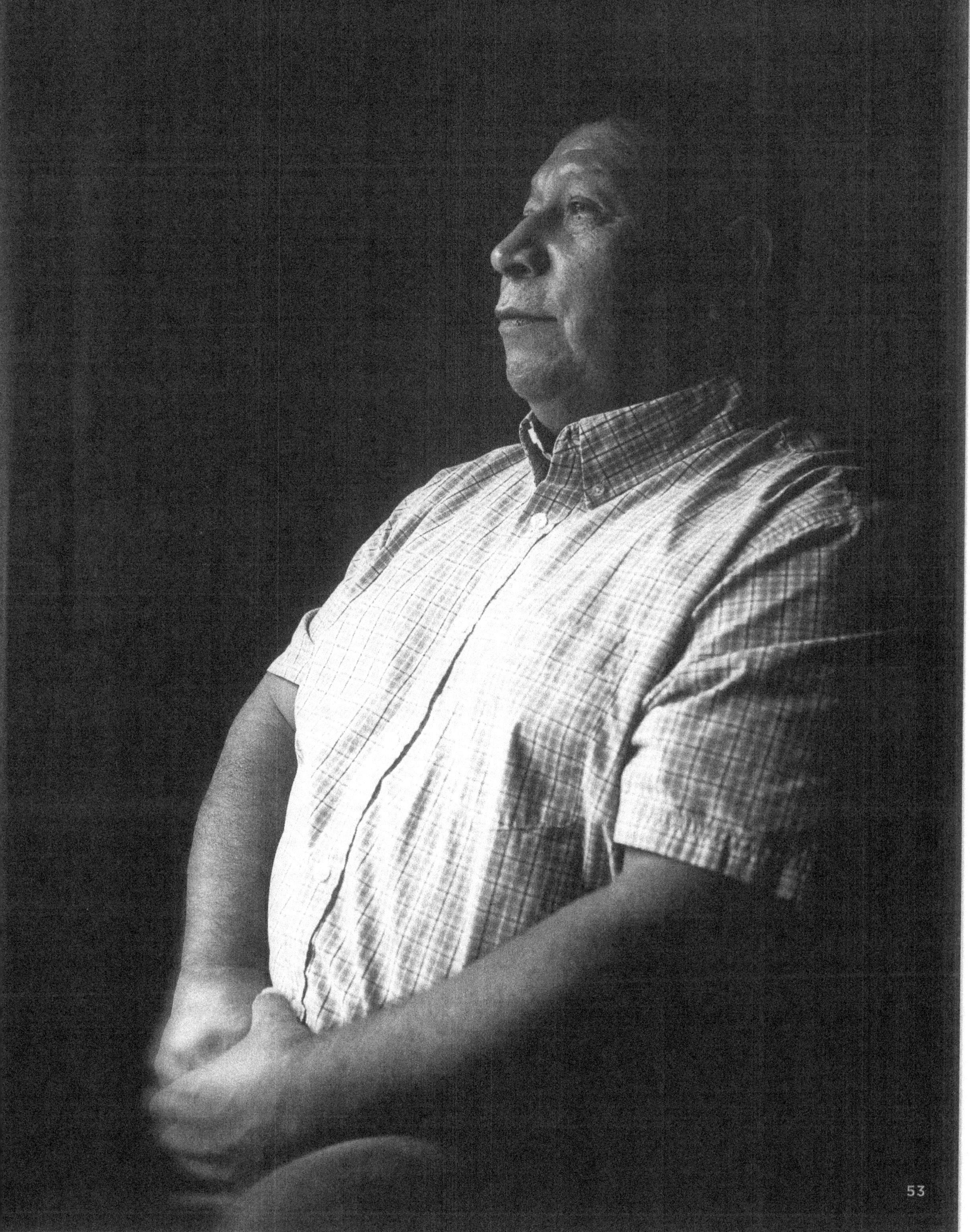

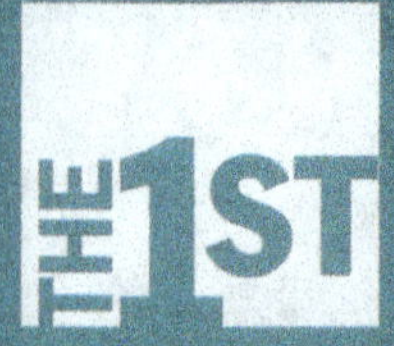

FIRST TO HIRE A
CERTIFIED **PEER
SUPPORT SPECIALIST**
IN MINNESOTA

In 2009, the Department of Human Services had an idea to train people with mental illness to work as peers in agencies, helping others who were struggling. They weren't exactly sure how to put the program together.

"And we said, 'Gee, we'd be very interested in supporting that.'"

MARY KAY MCJILTON, VICE PRESIDENT

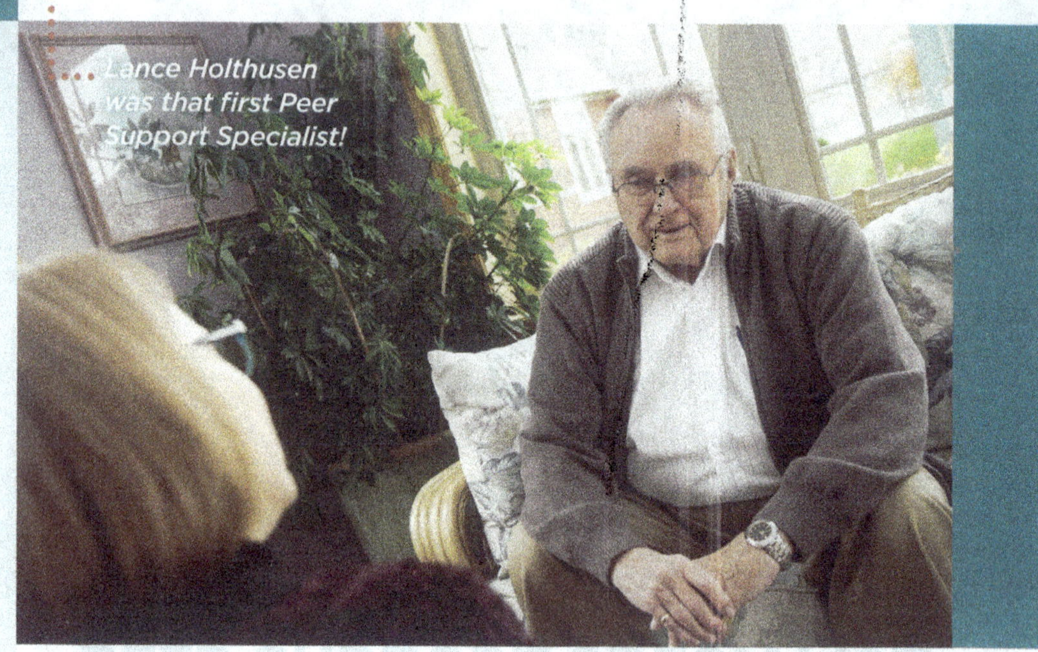
Lance Holthusen was that first Peer Support Specialist!

People in a crisis house are afraid to talk about what's going on. They're going to be judged again. They would say to me, "Who are YOU? A clinician?"

"No."

"What are you?"

"Well, they call me a Peer."

"What the heck does THAT mean?"

"Well, it just means I've done a few things that you'd probably under-stand. Some drinking issues. Some mental health issues. But why don't you talk about you?"

**LANCE
PEER SUPPORT SPECIALIST**

We had t-shirts printed up for all of the Peer Support Specialists at the fall conference.

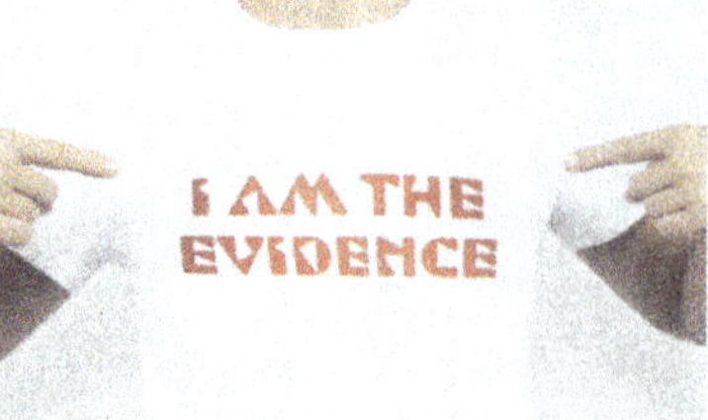

In other words, "*I'm standing in front of you. This is proof. It's possible to survive and get better.*"

GLENN ANDERSON, FORMER EXECUTIVE DIRECTOR

BY BEING WITH THE PEOPLE I SERVE, I'M JUST HAPPY BECAUSE THEY DON'T FEEL ALONE ANYMORE.

ALBERT, PEER SUPPORT SPECIALIST

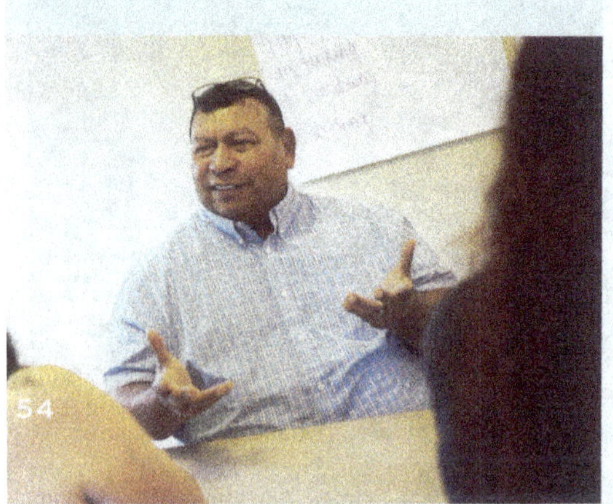

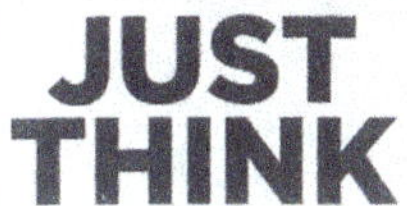

JUST THINK
AS MANY AS ONE IN FOUR AMERICAN ADULTS HAS A MENTAL ILLNESS.*
They are the people we love.
The people we count on.
The people who make us smile. 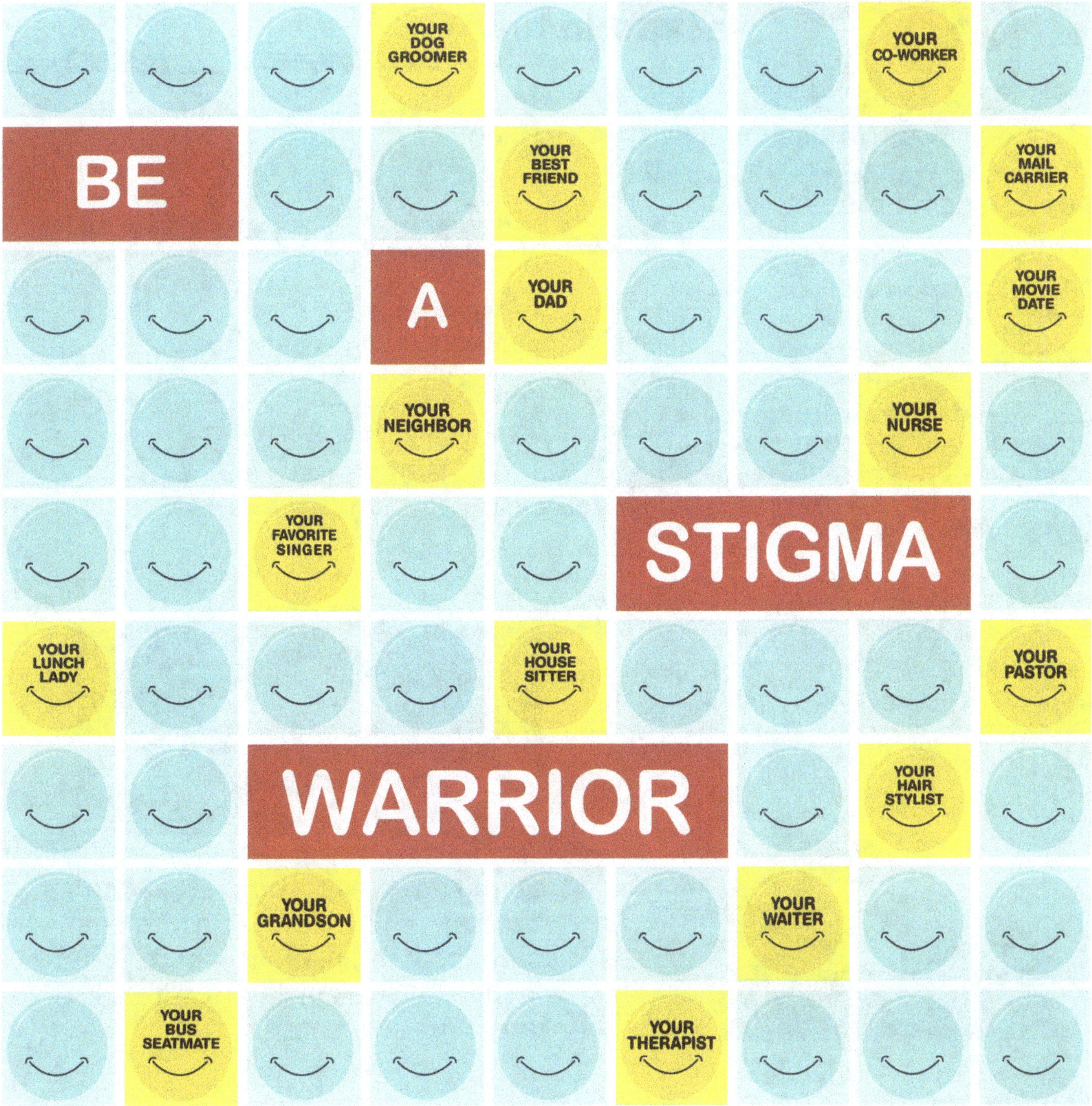
YOUR DOG GROOMER
YOUR CO-WORKER
BE
YOUR BEST FRIEND
YOUR MAIL CARRIER
A
YOUR DAD
YOUR MOVIE DATE
YOUR NEIGHBOR
YOUR NURSE
YOUR FAVORITE SINGER
STIGMA
YOUR LUNCH LADY
YOUR HOUSE SITTER
YOUR PASTOR
WARRIOR
YOUR HAIR STYLIST
YOUR GRANDSON
YOUR WAITER
YOUR BUS SEATMATE
YOUR THERAPIST
*Source: nami.org

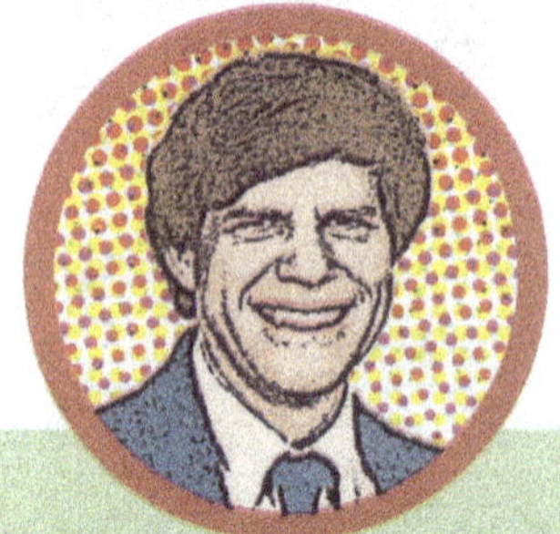

TIM BURKETT, FORMER CEO, REMEMBERS...

A Capital Idea!

IT WAS THE MID-1990s.
We wanted to create more programs for people with mental illness, but where could we get the funding?

Advocacy groups and trade groups normally went to the legislature on our behalf. But that process was slow-going and expensive.

I told a senator th at I wanted to bring in some homeless people and deaf people with mental illness to testify. And she said, "You'd better not bring any of them over here, Tim. You'll never get any money if you bring them over."

I brought them over anyway, and it was successful. It went well, and n ow it's common practice.

I'D GO INTO A LEGISLATOR'S OFFICE TO SEE WHAT PHOTOS THEY HAD ON THEIR DESK. IF THEY HAD A GRANDDAUGHTER, I'D ASK ABOUT HER.

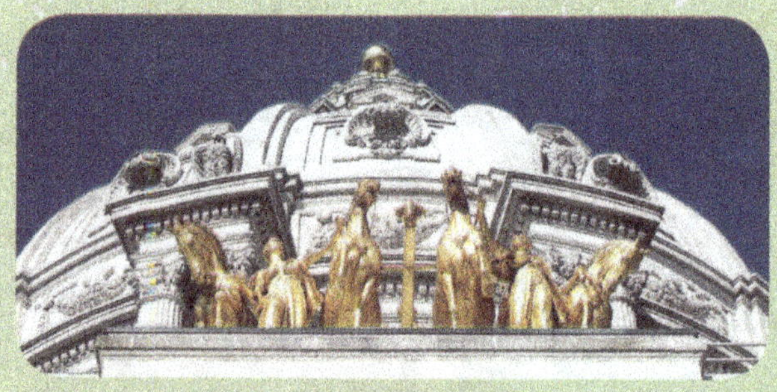

Some times legislators refused to see me, so I'd follow them into the bathroom to tell them our story. In the end, the legislators were the ones who advocated for us.

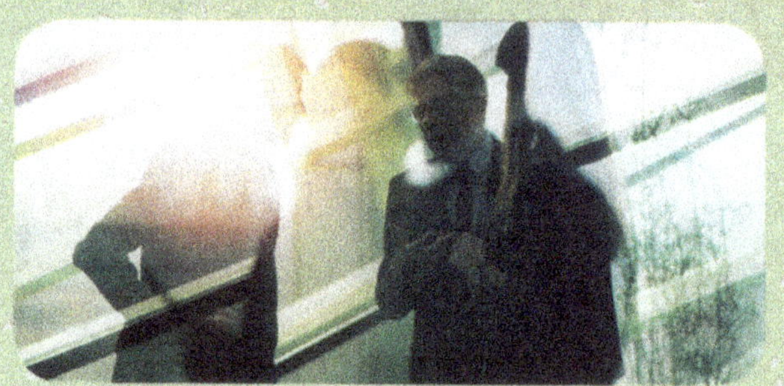

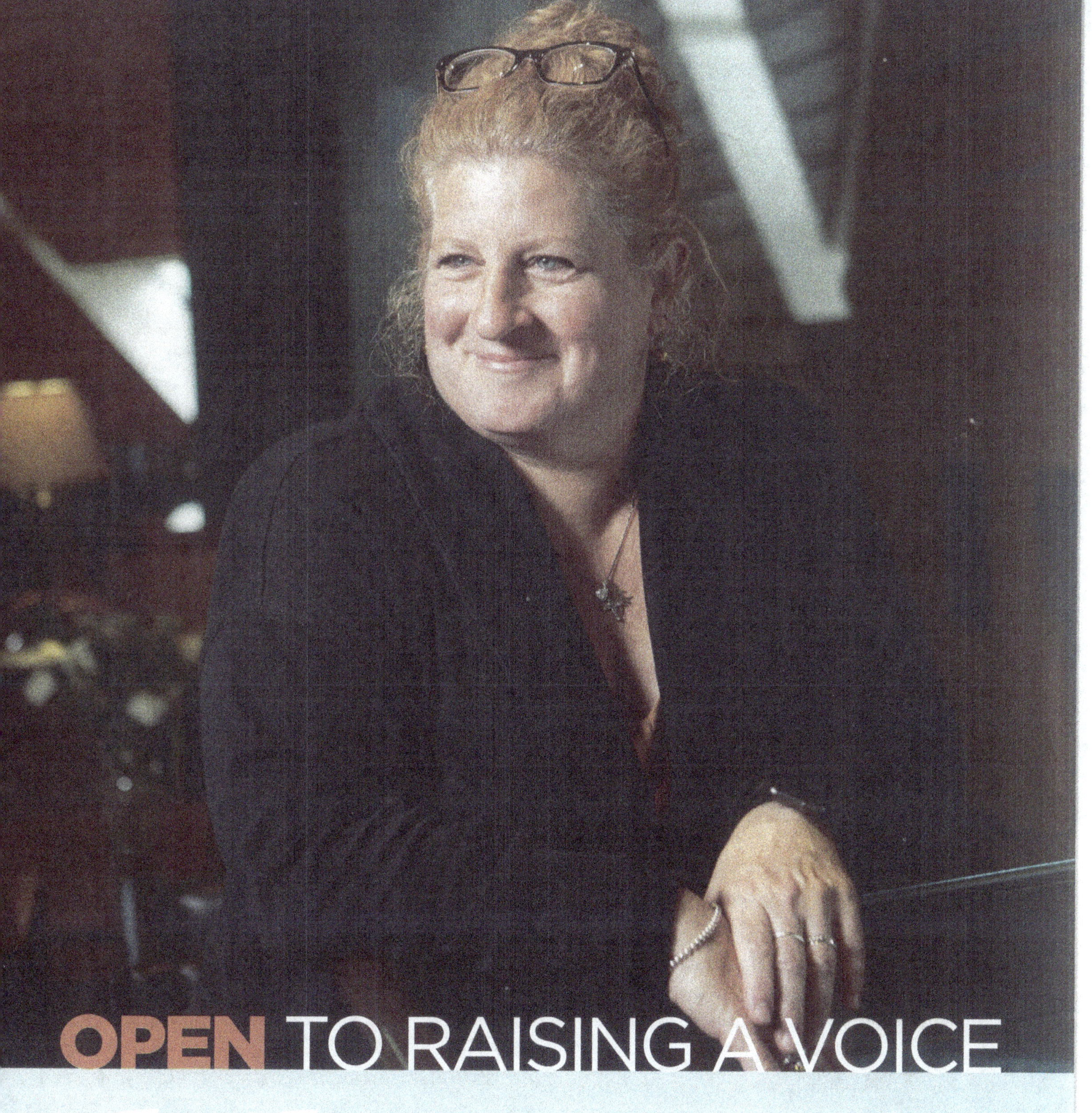

OPEN TO RAISING A VOICE

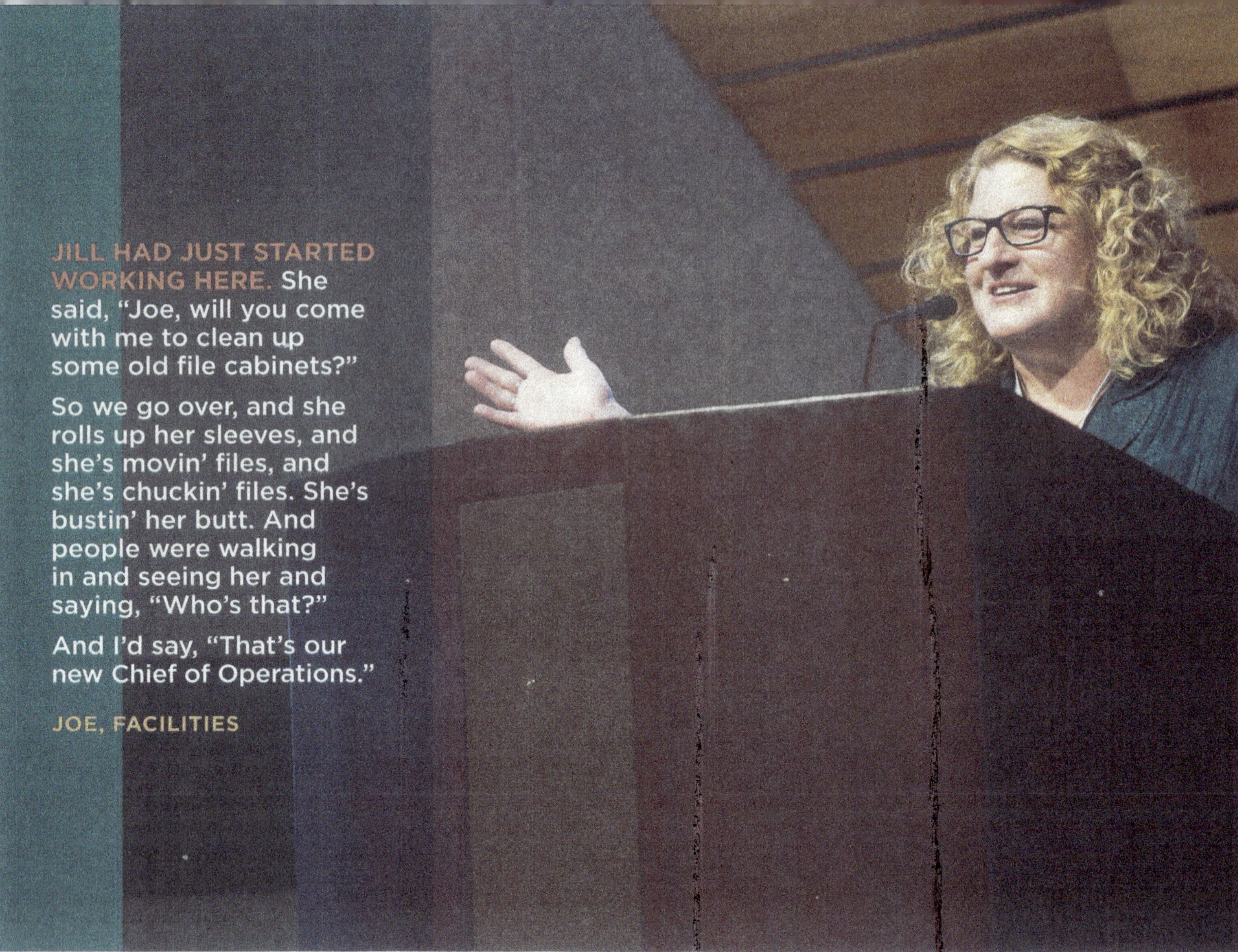

An excerpt from an interview with Jill

 You're making some pretty big changes in how People Incorporated approaches care. Do you ever worry you won't have the funding to see your vision through?

JILL: It doesn't keep me awake at night, because I think there's always a way. A way to get the money. A way to make service happen. It might not be immediately visible to me, but I believe barriers are meant to be jumped over.

Our growth curve in the last few years, partially, has been a little bit stronger and more stable, because we're looking at the business a little bit differently.

INTERVIEWER: *You just called your nonprofit a business.*

JILL: No doubt, we've got a very deep mission. But make no mistake, this is a business, 100 percent. And anybody who thinks that just caring alone is going to keep us a vibrant and strong business, is—short-sighted. There is no mission without a margin.

If I'm not continually innovating both at the client service level and in the manner we run our business, for sure I'll screw this up. And then the next 50-year anthology will be just one big, blank page of all that didn't go well, right?

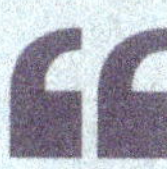

JILL IS THE PERFECT EVOLUTION OF—WELL, SHE'S JUST PERFECT. PEOPLE INCORPORATED HAS GOT A LOT OF HORSEPOWER. JILL IS RIDING A VERY STRONG HORSE, AND SHE KNOWS HOW TO RIDE.

GLENN ANDERSON, FORMER EXECUTIVE DIRECTOR

I personally owe a lot of gratitude to Jill for being that positive voice— someone I could go to. She's allowed me to become more culturally competent.

**SERGEANT JAMIE SIPES,
MENTAL HEALTH UNIT
ST. PAUL POLICE DEPT.**

People Incorporated is the largest community-based mental health nonprofit in the Upper Midwest. And we have a woman leading it. That's cool!

ALYSSA, PROGRAM SUPERVISOR

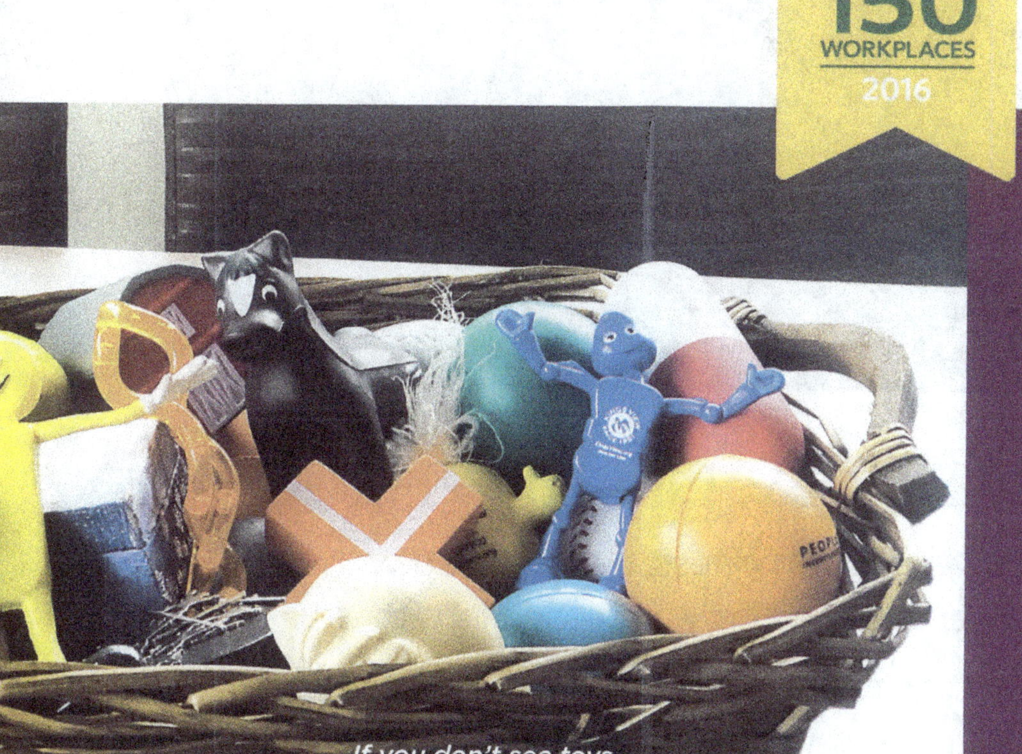

If you don't see toys, it's not Jill's conference table. Food for creative thought!

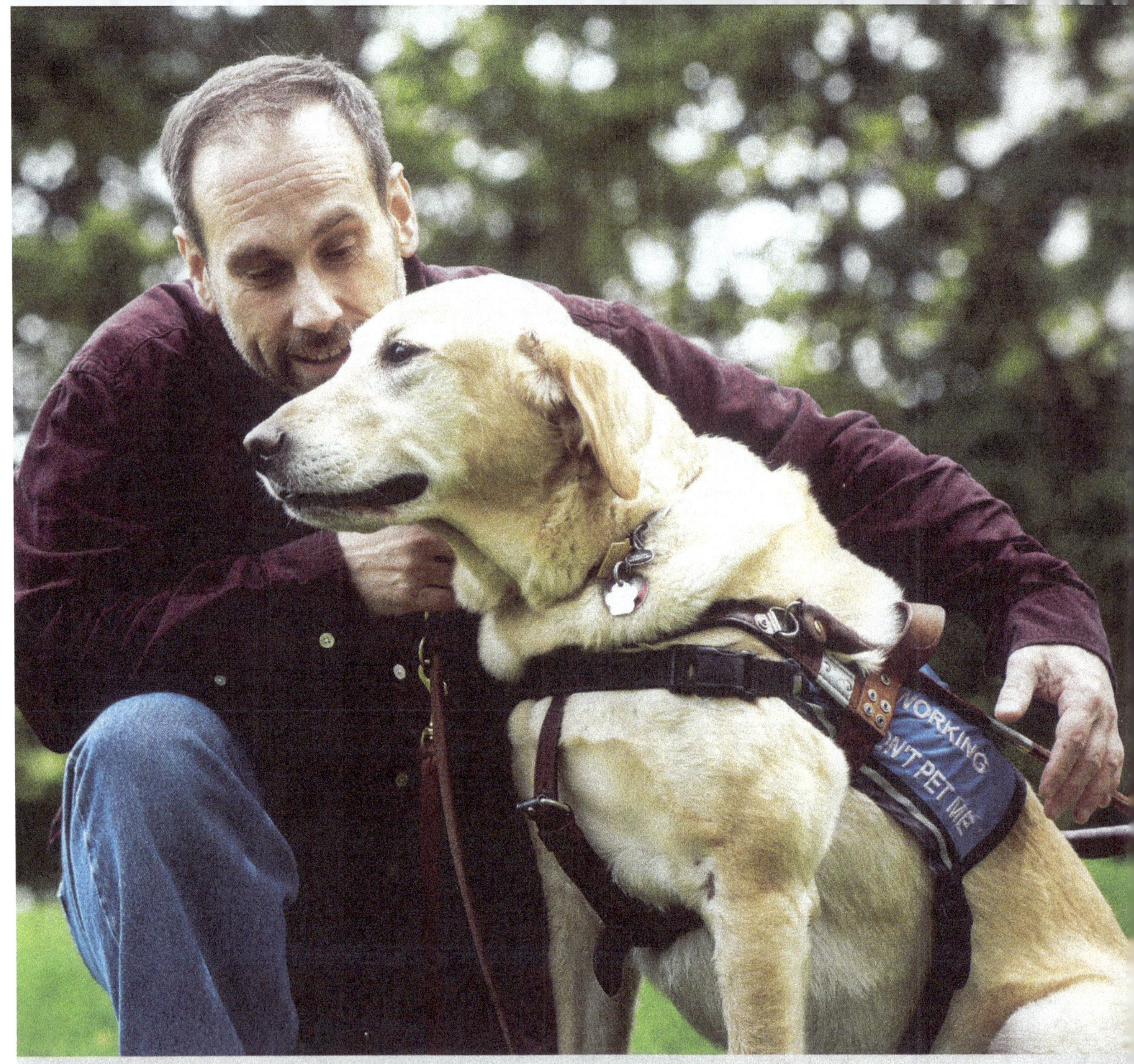

MEET KEVIN (and his guide dog Iliad).

Because of his blindness, he was filled with hatred for his eyes. So he poured bleach into them.

Today his world is filled with music. A composer and a pianist, he plays gigs all around the Twin Cities.

Cool stuff people said

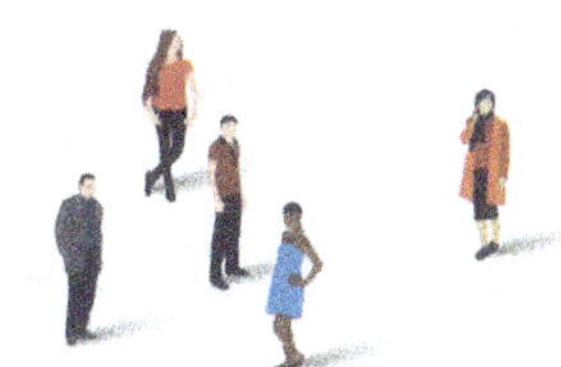

To create this book, we interviewed tons of people who gave us more memorable quotes than we could ever use. We've brought some delicious leftovers to share with you. Enjoy!

When I go to a new city, I don't usually look at the beautiful skyway. I'm looking along the highways to see how many camps they have. And what it's like to live under their bridges. I'm thinking, "Is there something I could be doing to help?"

KATIE, OUTREACH CASE MANAGER

MY ROLE, AS I SAW IT, WAS TO WORK WITH PEOPLE TO EVOKE THEM INTO LEARNING THAT THEY WERE PRECIOUS.

LANCE, PEER SUPPORT SPECIALIST

I MEAN, IT'S NICE THAT THIS BOOK IS BEING DONE. BUT IT'S MORE IMPORTANT THAT THE STUFF ACTUALLY HAPPENED, THAN TO GET IT WRITTEN DOWN.

**GLENN ANDERSON
FORMER EXECUTIVE DIRECTOR**

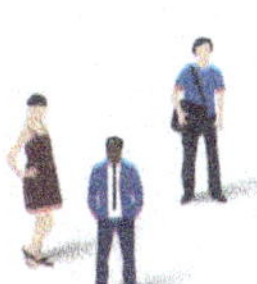
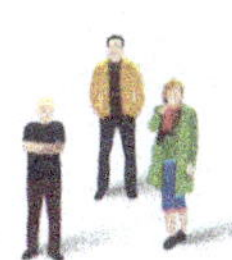
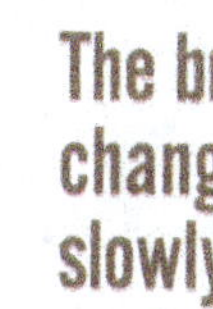

I myself battle with depression and anxiety. My depression tells me I don't care about anything, and my anxiety tells me I care too much about everything.

JOE, FACILITIES

All of us get depressed. We have addictions. We have fixed beliefs. It's just a matter of degree. Our folks are us, to the 10th Power.

JOAN, PROGRAM DIRECTOR

The breakthroughs and positive changes with clients happen slowly and far between. But it's such an incredible, soul-lifting experience that it sustains you.

**AMBER
PROGRAM MANAGER**

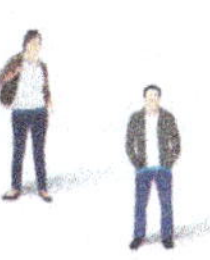
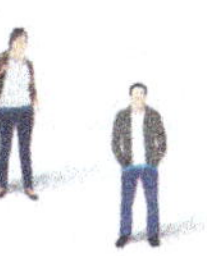

MENTAL HEALTH WORKERS DO NOT GO INTO THIS FIELD TO MAKE MONEY. IT'S A KICK-YOUR-BUTT-EVERY-DAY JOB. BUT ONE THEY LOVE.

BILL, COMMUNICATIONS DIRECTOR

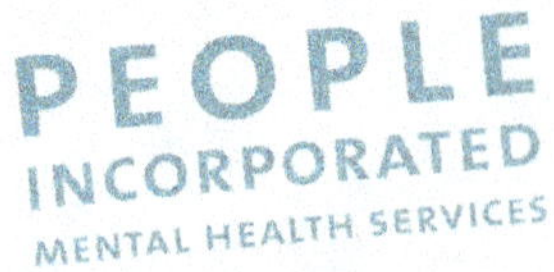

Dear Client,

How's it going? We're writing to let you know that we've been thinking about you a lot (for 50 years or so). And we thought maybe you'd like to hear about our plans for the next 50.

WE PROMISE, as always, to watch out for you.

WE PROMISE to keep educating ourselves. The more we know, the easier it is to invent new ways to make your life better.

WE PROMISE to help you manage what can be a very disabling illness in a world that isn't always friendly to it.

And **WE PROMISE** to help the community get to know you a little better. (Once they understand you, they'll love you as much as we do. So hang in there.)

Please take care of yourself, friend. You've got a dynamic disease, and things can get complicated pretty fast. If you could use some help, remember—we've got a whole bunch of people here who know you really well. We'll never abandon you.

Yours Very Truly,

People Incorporated

People Incorporated Mental Health Services

A Closing Thought

If there was a man in despair standing on the side of the road, our founders would offer him a sandwich, a cup of coffee, and a warm place to talk.

But they'd feel like they could do more.

Fifty years down the same road, a host of experts walk alongside this man. We ask him what kind of life he's trying to find. Someone puts a hand on his back to guide him. We help him climb walls and cross gullies.

And we feel like we can do more.

JILL WIEDEMANN-WEST, CEO

To the many keepers of
People Incorporated's oral history,
thank you for helping us turn
it into written word.

Creative Director, Writer: Carrie Maloney
Design: Barb Betz, Betz Design
Photography: Tony Nelson Photography
Project Manager: Bill Gray